Healing
the
Hurts
of
Childhood

MICHAEL HARDIMAN Ph.D

Revised and Updated. 2022
Formerly published as
Healing Life's Hurts.

To those who have the courage to change

Michael Hardiman Ph.D.
Nov 2023
Copyright © 2023 by Michael Hardiman
Published by
Paragon Books (Ireland) Ltd.
Galway Ireland

Contents

Foreword

I wrote this book in its original form 25 years ago. In the time since then there have been many improvements in the treatment of children and many younger adult readers will no longer identify with some of the content. I have made some minor changes to take account of these changes. At the time it was written many adults were recovering from seriously traumatic childhood experiences. It was a time when the revelations of the widespread sexual abuse of children with the Irish society at large, and more particularly at the hands of the Roman Catholic clergy had come to light. Since then, other revelations concerning the enslavement of young pregnant teenagers and the sale of their babies has added a shameful stain on our history. Thankfully a new generation of more caring adults and institutions leave these historical events in the past. There remains however a smaller group of people who still damage and abuse their children. The content of this book remains relevant to those who did experience these forms of trauma. And I do hope you will find much in it to enlighten you, even if it is to relate specifically to your own experience, but to help understand those less fortunate.

This is an optimistic book. Its optimism is, however, a guarded one. I believe that many approaches to healing and growth are marked by a naive romanticism about the true complexity of human nature. This naivete is reflected in many of the self-help books which adorn the shelves of most book shops. There is now a very large market for such books and this indicates a strong interest, among the reading public, in the areas of personal development, self-improvement and getting on better in life. Many self-help books, however, while worthy endeavours in themselves, often reflect simplistic and naive attitudes to the problems that they attempt to address.

We read in some that we can change our lives by deciding to think positively rather than negatively. In others we are encouraged to change by becoming more assertive in stating our needs and rights. Still others suggest that if we visualise ourselves in a better situation, or condition, it will come true. Whilst these and other approaches all have a certain validity, none are sufficiently comprehensive as a means of healing and recovery. At best, these approaches help people to be some what more effective in coping with their everyday lives. At worst, they provide us with a means of covering over the cracks with fancy mind-games that delay true recognition of our inner dilemmas and postpone our recovery. When reading this kind of material, I am reminded of Reiff's insightful comment that 'the cultivation of the self, taken as an ideal, is no guarantee against stagnation and despair'. Most people who have spent time, money and effort in trying to change their lives fundamentally realise what an enormous task it truly is. It is also important to recognise that there are important aspects of ourselves that are our genetic inheritance and these are of considerable importance in understanding how we react to trauma.

This book attempts to examine the areas of recovery and personal development in a way that gives due credit to the difficulties, challenges and opportunities that present themselves along the way. Its focus is limited to the specific subject of recovering from damaging experiences that occurred in the formative years of childhood. I believe that such experiences underlie many of the painful conditions that people experience in adult life. There are, of course, other painful and traumatic experiences that may have little or nothing to do with childhood. Losing one's job, the death of a spouse, the breakdown of a marriage, financial poverty and all the other varieties of circumstances that impinge on us at different points in our lives may have no connection to our childhood experience. It can be said, however, that the way in which we deal with these for better or worse - may be strongly related to what we learned and experienced as children.

While optimistic in outlook, this book does not under estimate the breadth and depth of human suffering. Nor does it advance the notion that healing and recovery is a simple process. Rather, its tone attempts to reflect the preciousness of human life and the belief that all of us have dignity, no matter how many layers of destructiveness to ourselves and/or others are wrapped around our souls. In this sense, my key themes here are those of suffering and its healing. As such, one of the areas that needs examination is the problem of suffering. I have devoted the first chapter to this subject.

CHAPTER 1
The Problem of Suffering

'Suffering does not ennoble the character sometimes happiness does.'
W. Somerset Maugham

Introduction

Over the past thirty years, I have been closely involved with the struggle faced by many people. I have seen individuals from all walks of life suffer varying degrees of internal turmoil. Others have suffered abuse at the hands of those close to them. Still others are trapped economically and socially, facing poverty and long-term unemployment, with little education and no saleable skills, their self-esteem crushed by feelings of having no worthwhile role to play in a world that seems to have dumped them. These problems and their effects on the human heart have all served to make me more aware of the experience of suffering, and the ways that people deal with it. This awareness has led me to make certain observations about the nature of suffering. These observations underlie much of the content of this book.

Some Comments on the Experience of Suffering

Firstly, some people's suffering is a legacy of having been damaged in childhood. During these formative years, the person is at his/her most vulnerable. Traumatic experiences are locked into the memory, sometimes out of consciousness, only to emerge in some form in adult life. Sometimes people will add new burdens of pain onto the old emotional scar tissue. Others will vent their pain on others and bring new suffering into the world. Recovering from such damage is in large part a matter of healing the wounds of the past and finding new ways of living healthily in the present. When this is done, the future takes care of itself.

Secondly, the experience of suffering plays a role in people's motivation to change. Most people who read books such as this do so out of inner turmoil. In general, they are looking for answers to the problems that they encounter. There are three categories into which these problematic experiences can be put.

Some people, for example, live a life filled with fear. They find it extremely difficult to speak up for themselves and hard to make friends. Others might look well on the outside, but carry deep inner sadness and loneliness. Still others are tense and anxious about themselves and their activities. This kind of suffering can best be described as emotional pain.

Then there are the spiritual and existential crises that come upon us at different times of our lives. For some, the whole of life seems to be a long journey filled with a yearning to find meaning. For others, there are intermittent struggles that involve confronting the significance of their existence in a world that often seems to trivialise their worth as human beings. This may be called existential struggle.

In addition, there is the suffering that eventually occurs for all of us when our physical bodies begin to decline, either through disease or the natural deterioration that leads to death. Certain people, however, are visited with long-term physical pain through disease or infirmity during what should be the healthier years of their lives. This experience can be accurately described as physical suffering.

These three areas of human suffering - emotional pain, existential struggle and physical suffering - are often intimately connected. On the one hand, it is a common enough occurrence to meet someone whose emotional pain leads to an existential/spiritual crisis that undermines their physical resources and leads to disease and sometimes to death. On the other hand, we can meet those whose physical deterioration leads to a spiritual/existential crisis which, if not resolved, can lead to an emotional breakdown. Then there are those whose existential/spiritual struggles lead to emotional and physical collapse. It is these experiences, either separately or in combination, that can lead people to search for a way forward toward a better life.

Thirdly, suffering is like mercury in a stream - it splits and flows in new directions, but never dissolves of its own accord. Suffering, therefore, afflicts those whose lives it touches. It continues from one generation to the next. Suffering parents cause turmoil, either directly or indirectly, to their children. Leaders who suffer bring tragedy to those whom they lead. Friends who suffer bring pain to those who care about them. When, therefore, we speak of healing and recovery, we are not only dealing with the individual's recovery; we are also making it possible for these positive changes to influence those around the sufferer, and those who are to come in future generations.

Fourthly, and related to the above, suffering can be a force for great good or great evil. The way that people cope with suffering largely determines whether or not it causes even more destruction in the world or whether it can have a positive outcome. I am concerned in this book with helping people see how their painful experiences can be turned into something of value. We know, for example, that some of the most beautiful creative acts have the experience of suffering at their roots. One only has to look at the beauty of Van Gogh's art, or listen to the haunting strains of a Chopin concerto, to appreciate the heartache out of which such priceless gifts to humankind have grown. On a darker note, however, we also see the cruelty and depravity that suffering can bring.

One of the more dramatic examples in this regard is the account of two ten-year-old boys who abducted a two-year-old toddler from a shopping mall, beat him, tortured him and killed him. When I read this story, I thought of my own son, who was almost eleven years old at the time. I tried to imagine how a mind so tender could partake in this kind of cruelty without having been already perverted by some experience. On further reflection, I remembered the birth of both my children, as they lay in their little cots amongst all the other new-born babies. Those two boy murderers were once, most likely, in a similar situation - all bundled up in swaddling clothes and warmed by the heat of the nursery. Which of us could walk among these little ones and predict those who would become so cruel and dangerous?

We now know that people who are violent have generally been exposed to violence at a young age. An important caveat here is to state that not everyone who is violated becomes violent. In fact, I would say that only a small minority do so. Similarly, others, who sexually molest children, are likely to have been molested themselves. These are not excuses for such behaviour. Rather, they are examples of the principle that the shadow side of human nature corrupts some of those who are its victims. And some of these victims then damage and destroy others. The paradox of human suffering is that it is the soil out of which grow the grotesque and the graceful, the loveless and the lovely, the cruel and the kind elements of human nature.

Some Comments on the Causes of Suffering

Certain basic assumptions with regard to suffering underlie the content of this book: 1. Most suffering is caused by people; 2. Most suffering is unnecessary; 3. Some people suffer greatly and/or cause others to suffer as a direct result of being emotionally damaged during childhood; 4. People can change the way that they deal with their own lives and the lives of others.

Most Suffering is Caused by People

There are two ways in which people act as agents for suffering and destruction. The first is the pain that we cause to others, either directly or indirectly. Directly, we can abuse and misuse others, we can destroy the souls of our children through psychological, physical and sexual abuse. We can directly harm others by releasing our anger at the world in attacking those weaker than ourselves, or taking pleasure in the misfortunes of others. We can also hurt others indirectly by driving wedges between people or by encouraging those within our sphere of influence to do harm to others. We can let our greed and fear prevent ourselves and others from relieving suffering, even if we had no part in causing it.

It is in this latter arena that we see the effects of collective responsibility for the suffering of others. It is by failing to stand out courageously against the injustice visited upon others by our peers, either politically or socially, that some of the greatest travesties against mankind have been wrought. Conformity is a powerful tool for both good and evil. Yet all collectives or groups are comprised of individuals. For such groups to function, there must be consent among the individuals within them. Each of us then either contributes or detracts from the collective's behaviour and, therefore, each of us bears some measure of responsibility for the group as a whole.

The second way individuals become agents for suffering is through the pain that we bring to ourselves. This usually has its roots in the first kind of suffering; namely, having been caused pain at the hands of others. The ways in which we cause ourselves to suffer most often involves undermining in some way the value of our lives. This self-destructiveness can take the forms of slow deterioration, by means of addictions, mental illnesses, and chronic stress through to the most tragic of all destruction - the taking of one's own life.

Most Suffering is Unnecessary

It is obvious that none of us can prevent the electrical storm that kills a young man while he shelters from the rain under an ill-fated oak tree. Nor can we see any reason why a child's blood cells begin to multiply aggressively, leading to a slow death from leukaemia. The bright and articulate human being who falls prey to conditions such as multiple sclerosis or Alzheimer's disease leaves all sensitive people with an awareness of the tragic and wasteful aspects of the human condition. These examples reflect 'necessary suffering', in so far as they are a part of being finite human beings who must eventually die.

Those who are left behind must also suffer the grief of loss and the sadness of lives cut short.

If, however, we were to quantify suffering, we would find that necessary suffering (those unavoidable painful experiences that come with being human, and for which there is no direct agent at work other than life itself) is far outweighed by the suffering caused by people to people and which could be avoided. Thus, most suffering is not a natural part of living, and is unnecessary. Some people suffer greatly and/or cause others to suffer as a direct result of being emotionally damaged during childhood

Benjamin Franklin once said that there are only two things in life of which we can be certain - death and taxes. While these are indeed enduring features of human life as we know it, there is something else that every adult can be sure of - we were all once children. What many do not realise, however, is that our experience of childhood shapes us in a myriad of ways and can influence us for good or for ill for the rest of our lives. There are many who do not believe this simple fact. Such people prefer to believe that when they became adults their logical, rational mind took over and provided a means of living life effectively. Life is seen as a series of problems to be solved and of challenges to be met. This logical approach is comforting in its simplicity, and yet greatly inadequate. There is too much desperation, turmoil and suffering in the world to allow us to believe that people are for the most part acting rationally. Something else is going on in the human experience.

Until recently, certain beliefs were commonly used to make sense of the unpredictability and complexity of the human story. The peaks of wonderful creativity and the passion of intimate love were considered as gifts from God, or the gods. The low points of evil and suffering were a legacy of fallen human nature, or the tricks of destiny, or the devil. These explanations, grounded in a religious view of the world, have offered comfort and a sense of order to humanity for most of our history. They have also produced a too ready acceptance of what is unacceptable, with the implicit belief that suffering is our fate.

More recently, with the advent and evolution of the physical and human sciences, a new optimism about the human condition developed. All problems could eventually be solved. People would live longer happier lives. People of good will would take power and use the world's enormous resources of intellectual and technological development to benefit mankind. However, despite significant changes and some advances in our ways of dealing with the world, new forms of human turmoil have grown alongside the changes that these developments have brought. In earlier times, people suffered and died of many illnesses that are now in the past. Now they die of new diseases. In earlier times, people suffered for their religious beliefs and the colour of their skin. Now more people die at the hands of violent sociopaths and crazed serial killers.

The modern world has not found the answers to human unhappiness in technology and social planning. People still abuse each other. Hatred takes new forms and wears new faces. Some think that we should return to the old ways of religious puritanism in order to solve these problems. To do this would only bring us back to the problems that were not solved when these ways of looking at the world were dominant. We would only succeed in exchanging our new problems for the old.

There is no single answer to the difficulties that face the human race. There will never be a time when our existence on this planet will be without strife. And yet each human being has the opportunity to make a difference, to make the world a better place to live in for himself and for those whose lives he touches. That many people will not, or cannot, do this means that there will always be a dark side to the human condition. This book is for those of us who want to change our lives and make a difference in our own corner of the world. It is not a treatise on political change, social awareness, or a global examination of the various systems that attempt to change the world. These are critically important in dealing with human destructiveness but are not the theme of this book. Rather, it is an examination of the way individuals come to terms with their own lives and relate to themselves and to others and to their environment.

In this context, the influences of childhood are of supreme importance in addressing the way that we live as adults, and if we wish to change, we have to examine these influences. A useful comment is made by Ernie Larsen, when he says 'What we live with we learn: what we learn we practice: what we practice we become.' The kind of people we become, whether we add to the burden of suffering or subtract from it, is there fore strongly based on what we have learned and experienced as well as on what we choose to do with these experiences.

People can change the way that they deal with their own lives and the lives of others

This assumption touches on one of the most contentious issues that has divided philosophers, scientists and religious thinkers over the centuries. As such, it could not be adequately discussed in detail without demanding the remainder of the book. Here, however, I wish merely to set out my position on the subject, with a brief explanation of what I mean by saying that people can change.

Firstly, change is difficult. It is not simply a matter of making up our minds to be different. Good intentions abound in the world, yet there are many blocks that prevent these intentions becoming an intrinsic part of our way of life. The human being is much too complex to be driven by a simple matter of a new resolution. Part of this complexity lies in the way that our lives are patterned by our past, and it is my belief that such patterns need to be understood before fundamental change can take place. Secondly, things are not always the way they appear. We can thank Freud for helping us to understand that human motivation is, in part, influenced by the dark and secretive passages of the unconscious mind. We need, therefore, to understand what lies beneath the surface of our everyday ways of living before we can realistically make any substantial changes.

Thirdly, the majority of human beings have some element of choice. Those of us who have a deep feeling of freedom in our lives are fortunate. We know that, for the most part, we can assert our will in order to do what we want. Such good fortune is a two-edged sword, for we can use our freedom to hurt or to heal. Others have more limited experience of freedom. Driven by basic instinct to survive, and finding little means to do so, life can seem greatly narrowed. Such people can feel completely at the mercy of their environment, with no room to manoeuvre. Still others are incapacitated and have little belief that anything they do makes any difference to their immediate situation. Change involves freedom. So it is important to examine how people can develop greater freedom in their lives. This can and does happen. I will discuss this area in more detail in Chapter 8.

Summary

We can now describe the elements involved in healing and changing one's life. Our first task is to examine the way that personality develops during the formative years of childhood. This includes the ways that we learn to deal with ourselves and the patterns of relating to others that are learned in the primary family relationships. These original strategies, of how to relate to ourselves and others, become for better or worse the map by which we chart our course through life. We will look specifically at those destructive patterns that emerge out of experiences within a dysfunctional family.

The second task is to examine how these patterns become habitual ways of coping with adult life. We will consider the ways in which these patterns affect our working lives and our relationships with others, including those intimate connections with our partners and children. We will also examine the way that these patterns affect our internal emotional and intellectual states, including the way that we experience and express our feelings, and the way that we view the world.

Once we understand how our formative years have affected us, and once we have identified the patterns of living that we carry from those experiences into our adult lives, then we can move on to the third task. This is the process of healing and change. This involves the elements of healing emotional damage, learning to think differently, changing our behaviour, and developing our spirituality. The remainder of this book is devoted to explaining these tasks in detail.

CHAPTER 2
The Family

Introduction

I stood looking up at John. His big brown eyes dilating, muscles tensing and his laboured breathing all told me that he was fighting to control his impulse to hit me. He didn't smell too good as his chest drew nearer to me. I, for my part, dressed in professional garb, pen in hand and glasses slightly forward on my nose must have looked an easy target for his growing rage. I held his eyes and spoke softly, hoping to ease his anger while coping with my own fear. For John, I was representing all the people in his life who had made him feel inferior. His mother, who was too emotionally exhausted to respond to the young child growing up too quickly for her amidst the deprivation of her family. His father, who never took any interest except to beat him when he felt like it. Teachers, who gave up on him when he showed no interest in his schoolwork and who humiliated him as a means of punishing him for acting up and causing trouble. The police, who chased him when he stole cars and treated him roughly when he was caught. And now here he was, on a training programme for young dropouts, having to listen to another one of these know-alls with their university education and fancy language.

Speaking softly, I told John that I knew he wanted to hit me and that I knew it wasn't easy for him to have to listen to what I was saying. I told him that I would prefer if he didn't attack me, that we could find a better way of sorting things out and that I was on his side. I sensed his rage gradually easing, as I suggested that he go for a smoke and think about what he would like to say. The crisis over, I went back to the remainder of the group to continue working on the project in hand.

Michael sits across from me, with his legs crossed and his piercing, intelligent eyes watching me carefully, as he analyses what I am saying. A successful medical consultant with a sharp mind and a successful practice, he is tormented with self-doubt and insecurity. His stress level and compulsive need to bury himself in work are causing a great deal of inner turmoil and a breakdown in his relationships with others, particularly with those close to him. He is impatient and unreceptive to what he is hearing. He wants a quick fix so that he can get on with his life. Toward the end of the session, his frustration with me grows, but he keeps it all inside, not wanting to appear rude or angry with me because I don't have an easy solution for what is in fact a complex problem.

These two people are a world apart in terms of outward appearance. They suffer, however, from a similar complaint. Both their personalities and ways of living in the world are still being strongly influenced by their experiences of growing up in dysfunctional families. Each has been destructively affected in the three dimensions of personality - their cognitive, emotional and social development. John is cognitively impaired. His attention span is short and he cannot concentrate for any reasonable length of time. His thinking is concrete and he doesn't cope well with the world of ideas and inner imagination. Growing up in an environment which lacked stimulation, colour and conversation, he doesn't reflect on problems: in other words, he doesn't know how to think. Michael, on the other hand, is cognitively over-compensating. His early environment lacked in security and love, while at the same time telling him that to be well educated and professional was the only way forward in life. He now functions almost completely in the world of ideas. As a result, he is a very thorough and efficient doctor, his scientific mind grappling with the minutiae of his particular area of specialisation. These skills are not helping him in the world of personal relationships, and his tendency always to convert experiences into intellectual problems means that he is badly equipped to learn about the aspects of life that are not intellectual.

Both are emotionally impaired. John's emotional life is like a blunt instrument. His main feeling is that of anger, and his focus is on taking out this aggressiveness on the world. To feel pity is to be a 'softy' and to lose respect. Tender feelings are rare, and only sometimes sneak in behind his angry defensiveness. Sex for both John and Michael is mainly a matter of physical pleasure and release. John has little or no insight into himself and blames others for his bad feelings. Michael, on the other hand, is unable to relax into the tenderness offered by his partner. To do so would open up the feelings of insecurity and helplessness that lie deep inside.

Socially, John is a reject. The only place he feels socially at home is with his gang. These all share a similar story: a group of young men who are physically strong, bored with life and unable to create useful, constructive activities for themselves. Consequently, they are at war with society in general. Their social skills are minimal. Because of their physical strength, they are able to do burdensome work that requires little intellectual skill. Yet such work is becoming scarce as human labour is replaced by robotics and by the world of technology. They have little prospect for fulfilment or development within present-day society.

Michael is a social success. He has money, respectability and a job that challenges him. His prestige is a mask he wears in order to fulfil his rather desperate need for affirmation. No matter how well he does, and no matter how much money he makes, he is still unhappy. His social contact with others is fraught with the need to prove his worth. This comes across as arrogance, which makes it difficult for him to make real friends. Most of his social contact is with others who play the same game as himself; all trying to establish a pecking order of success, which leaves them with a gnawing emptiness and a frustrated desire to be able to get beyond the social games into real contact with others.

These stories serve as a useful starting point for our discussion of the effects of childhood experience on adult lives. Three areas have been mentioned: cognitive and emotional development, and social learning. A great deal of personality formation is laid down in these areas before the age of ten. When this formation is dysfunctional and destructive, the way is set for certain patterns of relating to oneself and the world to become reinforced and rigid during adolescence. These patterns then become the map for life that a person brings into adulthood.

Conversely, when the primary influences on a child's life are positive, these become the foundation for identity building in adolescence and thus a positive map for adult life. Naturally, there are exceptions to every rule, and some people who have had very positive childhood years lose their way during adolescence. Similarly, some children who have suffered in their formative years are exposed to sufficient positive influences during adolescence to counteract much of the effects in a way that leaves them well prepared for adult life. These situations are, however, relatively rare. I will discuss the three areas of development in more detail later in this chapter. Before doing so, I wish to explore the major factors that provide much of the influence on a child's development.

These influences are found primarily through the child's experiences within the family, the school and his or her peer group. There is a gradual change in the power of each of these influences as childhood progresses. In the early years, the family is of foremost importance; then the experience of school begins to take effect; and by the age of twelve, the peer group begins to take over as a major factor. This chapter examines the crucial role of the family in building an individual's personality.

The Family

Until very recently, the vast majority of people in western society grow up in what is called a nuclear family. This means that the powerful influences on a child's early development lie in the hands of two people: their father and mother. In earlier times and in some different societies today - such influence was less concentrated because many adults had access to, and responsibility for, the rearing of children. The advent of the industrial revolution saw a major change in the early experience of children, as well as the development of cities with vast concentrations of people in small areas. More specifically, the biological unit of parents and their offspring became the norm of society.

This development has left children in a precarious position, because so much now depends on the qualities of their parents in terms of how they treat their children. When such treatment is positive, the nuclear family provides a great deal of protection and love for developing young ones. When the treatment is negative, the nuclear family becomes a private place of suffering, where few outsiders can intervene. Although we may be at the stage where the nuclear family is breaking down, where grandparents are taking more responsibility for children, where couples no longer stay together for the sake of the children or out of economic necessity, there is as yet no clear alternative to the nuclear family.

It is, therefore, important to the theme of this book to examine the influences of the nuclear family in terms of child development. The notion that early childhood experiences, both positive and negative, have powerful long-term effects on the way that people function is a central theme of this book. It would be simplistic, however, to suggest that these experiences are not profoundly influenced by the value system that operates in a society at a given time. Thus, the manner in which a family operates is to some extent a reflection of the society in which that particular family exists. Let us look at some examples. Certain cultures carry a very repressive ideology that sees women as inferior to men. A family in this culture will treat boys very differently than girls. It is far more likely that girls reared in such families will experience a lot of fear of men as well as limited confidence, low self-esteem and a passive, submissive role in relation to social issues.

Changes in modern western society are also having profound effects on the way that families function. One of the more recent trends is leading to what Robert Bly calls the 'fatherless society'. More and more often we see that marital breakdown leads to the impoverishment of the couple and in particular the marginalisation of men. More specifically, in leaving their role as partner to the woman, many men lose their role as parent to the children. This social reality is profoundly affecting children's development, as well as creating new social problems that in turn will affect the following generations. (This phenomenon is examined in more details in another book of mine: "Ordinary Heroes")

Other aspects of social change do not directly affect the nature of the relationships within the family, and yet can prove very influential in the experience of children. An obvious example is poverty. When most people in a society are financially impoverished, then there is little stigma in being poor. Children going to school with patched clothes, third hand school books and small lunch boxes are all, so to speak, in the same boat. If, however, a large number of children are in families that are relatively well off, they will have good clothes, extra goodies for lunch, money for the shop, nice bicycles, computer systems iPads smart phones and the like. In this context, a child from a poorer background can find himself marginalised, or different from the majority, and this can lead to shame, self-consciousness and many other self-esteem problems that have little to do with his relationships within the family. Economic issues therefore, also affect early experience.

Social, economic, and political realities affect the way in which families function, and in certain situations political and social change need to precede changes in family systems. This book is, however, limited to discussing the internal workings of the family and must leave the wider political and social issues for another time. For whatever reason, then, there are two categories of families: those that provide the necessary care and treatment of children so that they can emerge from childhood well equipped to live a fulfilled life in today's world; and those that create such problems for children that their personalities become damaged. I will call these categories healthy families and dysfunctional families respectively.

Healthy Families

What is a healthy family? On the surface, this seems a rather simple question, but like most important questions, the answer is more complex than it first appears. Health is a relative term. In other words, we could say that a person living on the streets in Calcutta is healthy in comparison with the others in his or her community, but is unhealthy in relation to people in a different social context

I consider a healthy family to be one which prepares a child to live in a balanced, wholesome way within the culture to which he or she belongs. This approach includes the two aspects of psychological well-being and cultural relevance. (I am aware that in certain societies it is impossible to fulfil both of these conditions at the same time.) Despite the powerful influences of ideology that suggests that human activity must always be accepted if it is the norm of a culture, there is no doubt in my mind that certain cultural practices run counter to human well-being.

For the purposes of this book, the main focus is on how families within western society operate. This means that a healthy family is one which influences a child in such a way that he is able to take on the challenges and opportunities of modern western society - a difficult and complex task. In a different era, a child could emerge from a family with only rudimentary education, one basic skill, limited abilities to communicate, little self-knowledge, and still be able to live effectively within that society. Today, such a person would find himself on the margins, open to very subtle and sophisticated messages from marketing strategists, through the world of television, and social media, financially impoverished, living in a small space surrounded by others just like himself (there are, of course, rare exceptions to every rule). The effects of these and all the other pressures of modern society have a crippling effect on psychological functioning, leading to a variety of problems. The vast increase in prescription medication usage for mood disorders and mental distress is clear evidence of the growing levels of personal anguish afflicting huge numbers in modern society. These problems in turn sometimes result in self-destructive activities, including addictions, family violence or some other form of criminality.

Modern society demands a great deal from the people living within it. Many are ill-prepared within their family of origin to take on the task of living in such a complex world. Taking these demands into account, the following are, in my view, the hallmarks of a healthy family. This list is not exhaustive, but I believe it covers the important areas:

1.serenity; 2. security; 3. respect; 4. affectionate love; 5. understanding; 6. discipline; 7. flexibility; 8. fun; and 9. equality.

With a moment's reflection, you will realise that these refer in large part to the emotional atmosphere within the family unit.

Serenity

Serenity refers to the peaceful atmosphere within the home. In general, this will be to a great extent a reflection of the internal emotional state of the parent or parents, and the way that they relate to each other and their children. Naturally, there will always be situations that occasionally disrupt the day-to-day running of the family. It can be said, however, that healthy families generate a sense of consistency in the way that things occur. Many different kinds of family units exist. Some reflect a lot of order, such as consistent mealtimes, routine homework times and an agreed television and screen time. Other families are more varied and diverse in their approach. This variety does not mean that serenity is absent; children adapt to certain fluctuations in everyday experience as long as they do not feel under threat by them. Consistency is then the key element here, as this allows for a great deal of differences in the way the family is run.

Security

Security refers mainly to the quality of the relationships between the parents and children. Children feel secure when they have a sense that the relationships within the family will not change drastically from one day to the next. A child's relationship with their parents, for example, needs to reflect a bond of loving concern that continues to grow and develop over the years. In families where a couple live together with the children, the relationship between the parents is seen by the child as an enduring bond. This gives the child a sense of security in knowing that Mum and Dad are at the head of the family and in general are going to look after him. Separation and divorce damage this security, but a great deal can be done to protect the child from the worst effects by a commitment from the parents to continue co-operating with each other in the tasks of parenting their children. This can happen even when their personal relationship has ended or changed from a marriage to some other form of relationship, one that can range from friendship to a mutual respect of their differences. Children can experience more security from separated parents who cooperate with each other than from those who stay together and are in conflict most of the time.

Respect

Mutual respect is a hallmark of a healthy family. This respect has many dimensions. The respect of the parents for each other means treating each other as people of worth and value in their own right. It means respecting the need for each person to hold individual values and aspirations, as well as not using each other in a way that is harmful to either. Similarly, respect for the individuality of each child means giving value to the growing unique identity of that child. It means allowing children to have their own views of the world and a right to a private self. It means respecting the physical and emotional boundaries of the child and helping him or her to grow in appreciation of who they are It also means generating a sense of bodily integrity which is reflected in letting children dress privately when they wish to do so and communicating that their bodies belong to them, and are not abused in any way through violence or sexual molestation.

Affectionate Love

Affectionate love for children is a high calling. It requires deep commitment to the child's developmental needs, which grow through stages, from utter helplessness and reliance on the parents' care, to mutual respect and friendship. In a healthy family, the parents grow and change in their relationship with their children as the children develop. These changes are underscored by an emotional attachment to the unique individual who is gradually forming an identity of their own. It is reflected in a concern for their welfare at all the stages of childhood. It is supportive, comforting, challenging and at times confrontational. The course of the relationship is marked out by consistent experiences of quality companionship and shared activities.

Children who grow up in such families have many special memories of contentment and happiness, of special times when they were given individual time of sharing activities with their parents, of fun-filled incidences where they could laugh together and of other times when they could bring their hurts into the presence of the parent and find solace and healing. When we use the above description as a benchmark for healthy love, it becomes clear that an enduring myth in modern society is that parents love their children. It appears that most parents are affected deeply by their own upbringing and the social consensus in this regard. It has therefore become a taboo in our culture to admit that certain parents really do not love their children. We would prefer to idealise the bonds between parents and children rather than honestly deal with what is going on inside the four walls of some family homes. Many parents are themselves emotionally impaired, to the extent that their capacity truly to love their children is considerably compromised. The often-held view that once we look after the physical needs of children, don't actively do them any harm, and let them get on with growing up, is a sufficient form of healthy love is neither accurate nor acceptable.

Understanding

I recently watched one of the now fashionable film comedies based on family issues. Like all good comedies, it had a serious theme. One of the older children in the programme nicely summarised the reality of life for many children. In the context of a family in crisis, she told her friend that it struck her as ironic that people had to have a license for owning a dog or driving a car, and yet it was readily acceptable for anybody to bring a human being into the world and effectively shape its life for good or ill. For most of us, the hugely responsible and complex task involved in becoming an effective parent is left almost completely to ourselves. Children in the modern world spend an average of fifteen years in full-time education without learning anything about the most responsible job of adult life - that of being a parent. This enormous gap in our preparation of young people for life has its roots in our historical understanding of childhood.

It is only relatively recently in historical terms that the Western world has recognised that childhood is a special stage of life. Up to then children were considered little adults. The fact that childhood was a formation period where experiences were indelibly inscribed in the personality lay unrecognised. Today, the incredible complexity of the human mind is an accepted fact. That childhood is a special stage of life is also recognised. In healthy families, there is an understanding of the child as a human being in formation. In such families, there is no expectation on the child to become an adult before their time. There is allowance for dependency on parents and there is room for gradual progress toward independence. Parents in healthy families take time to learn about child development. They do not assume that the biological facility to bear children equips them to be good parents. Healthy people, in general, continue to learn and grow throughout their lives. When they become parents, they bring this openness to learning into their new role, and recognise its fundamental importance. They thus learn to understand their children.

Control

Imagine sitting in an aircraft on a transatlantic crossing flying at 31,000 feet, at a speed of 500 miles per hour. You are relaxing after watching the in-flight film, and perhaps dozing off. Then you see a flight attendant scurrying up the aisle toward the cockpit with a frantic look on her face. She talks to her colleagues and you see them talking to each other furtively, all wearing the same expression of concern and controlled panic. You begin to feel the fear rising, very imperceptibly at first, just a butterfly feeling in your stomach and a slight increase in heartbeat. Then you notice the plane beginning to change direction. It's beginning to dive. Now your fear begins to grow. Suddenly the soothing voice of the captain comes over the intercom. He tells you not to worry, that the plane is descending to avoid turbulence. Still worried, you call the flight attendant to ask if there is something wrong, that you noticed her seeming perturbed. She apologises and tells you that she dropped her engagement ring into one of the food trays. You breathe a sigh of relief and go back to your own thoughts. The crisis is under control.

This little cameo tells us something about what it feels like to be at risk when we have no control. Healthy families exude a sense that the people 'in the cockpit' are capable, competent and know what to do in the running of the family. There are few, if any, scenes of hysteria. There is a calm approach to family issues and conflicts. People are listened to and their opinions are sought when decisions that affect them are to be made. Of course, some of these decisions may not suit everyone, but at least they know that their opinions have been taken into account. Parents in healthy families are authoritative. They realise that it is their joint responsibility to create an environment where people live safely and happily together. They make rules based on respect for each family member and implement these in a caring, but firm, way.

Discipline

Closely related to control is the place of discipline in the family. Discipline refers to setting boundaries for behaviour, and the use of authority. In order to implement it. For children to grow into healthy well-adjusted adults they need the stability and safety of strong external authority in their early years. This is because the do not have the internal structure by which to regulate their own behaviour. In time these external rules are internalised and the child is above to develop self- discipline which is an absolutely essential part of mature adulthood. Currently there is a naïve failure to recognise that establishing firm external boundaries for children is essential to their healthy development

Flexibility

Although control is a necessary part of a healthy family, it needs to be balanced with flexibility. This means that the family system changes and evolves as the people within it develop and learn. One of the key areas of control within the family is the set of rules (sometimes unspoken and un conscious), by which the family operates. These rules are generally understood by everyone in the family. They can be categorized as rules concerning how people relate to each other and what feelings or behaviours are forbidden or encouraged. Within a healthy family, there is a good deal of flexibility and adaptability in how these rules are created and applied. Thus, for example, old rules about certain behaviours can change when it becomes clear that they are too stifling or unreasonable. Others can become obsolete because the individuals have grown beyond the need for them. A useful comment in this regard is that the rules that exist within a healthy family grow out of the relationships. The relationships are not defined and confined by the rules. When this approach is taken, then no rule becomes written in stone. I will discuss the devastating results of rigidity and legalistic authoritarianism in the section on dysfunctional families.

Fun

Healthy families are characterised by fun. People within such a family, for the most part, enjoy each other. Naturally, there will be moments of conflict and certain children will get on better with each other. One of the characteristics of people who get on well is the amount of laughing they do together. I am not discussing the nervous, tension relieving laughter that has a slight edge of hysteria. Rather I am referring to the joyous laughter of people who love each other. A parent will catch the eye of his or her child especially when something silly or funny has happened; their eye contact will speak volumes and both will spontaneously start to laugh. Or a child will be in the throes of some disagreement and the parent will tell him to 'chill out' and they end up wrestling on the floor. Spontaneous enjoyment is, then, an intrinsic part of a healthy family.

Equality

Every child is unique. Healthy families recognise this. Children are treated as equals. They are given equal time and attention. No one is marginalised or treated as the problem child, and similarly no one is consistently selected out for special attention. This is true even when there is a natural affinity between certain children and their parents. Some children, for example, are born with a temperament that makes it easier to relate to them. They may be placid and easy going. They make fewer demands and recover from conflict more quickly. Others are more inclined to become cranky when they don't get their way. They are stubborn and more difficult to satisfy. Healthy families allow these differences and compensate for them. Parents don't live in a continual reaction to the more assertive children, recognising that such strength can be channelled into wholesome activity and can be a real bonus to preparing the child for the tough world of adult life. Similarly, they don't ignore and take for granted the quieter child.

'Equal but different' is the motto of a healthy family. This is also reflected in the relationship between parents. It has been a feature of all human societies heretofore that men and women take different roles in the structure of both their families and their society/tribe. More recently, in the modern world, the differences have become less profound. Control over fertility, economic independence and shifts in values concerning the roles that are acceptable for both men and women all lead to greater levels of equality between the sexes. In consequence much conflict has now arisen as various positions are taken concerning any consideration that there may be real difference between the sexes. The current 'culture war' is partly a fight about the notions of gender and sex. This is unfortunate, because it suggests that equality is based on sameness. That is an unwelcome outcome. I prefer to believe that as we are all human we merit respect and value on this basis alone. In healthy families the partners can take very different roles without undermining each other's value. Similarly, the vast differences that can occur between children are not used as a justification to treat one as better than the other.

I can imagine some readers raising their eyebrows with what I've written so far. It is a telling sign of our times that to describe a healthy family in the terms above can be met with a certain disbelief. This is because in the western world, at least, such families are becoming a rare phenomenon. High level of divorce is leaving many children bereft of fathers. Even in intact families so many children are largely reared in childcare facilities because economic necessity forces both parents to work full time. Add long stressful journeys to places of work cutting into whatever time is left for parents who often arrive home exhausted with just enough time left to feed the kids and get them to bed, only to do it all again the following day. And that's when everything is going well!.

We have almost given up on the prospect of such families being the norm, rather than the exception, resulting in rampant cynicism about family life. There is a sound basis for such cynicism. Many commentators believe that the modern-day family is in crisis, and they are right.

The discussion of healthy families should not suggest that the way forward is to return to the kind of idealistic utopian notions often displayed in the sentimental 'little house on the Prairie.' That social model often hid a very different story of family life. In my own society, the power of the Roman Catholic Church was almost complete in the way that people were told to live their lives. One of the well known clichés in this regard was that 'the family that prays together stays together'. The moral value was, based on staying together no matter what. This led to a great deal of dishonesty and hypocrisy. Family units torn by strife and turmoil, where children grew up terrified and damaged, were acceptable as long as they could project a good living image to the outside world. Others, who did the decent thing and split up rather than further damage each other or their children, were treated as pariahs.

The walls of denial, so well-constructed throughout the centuries, are breaking down. We are beginning to see that behind the exterior presentation there are many families that are sick and dysfunctional. These families create damaged children, who grow up into damaged adults, who marry each other and create new dysfunctional families.

All the major roles that people play in life are dramatically influenced in their family of origin. We learn, in that microcosm of society, how to be a man or a woman, how to be a mother or a father, what childhood means, how to function in society. The family is the. building block of society and essential for its survival. Sick societies are the product of sick families. It is to this topic that we now turn.

Chapter 3.
Dysfunctional Families

The word 'dysfunctional' is now fashionable, at least within the 'psychologized' areas of society. When it is used to refer to a family it means that the family does not function in a healthy way. It does not operate in such a way that the people in it, both parents and children, find within its confines the experiences that lead to emotional health, creative productivity, high self-esteem and a love of life.

I am impressed with Warren Farrell's comments (in his book The Myth of Male Power) on the use of the word 'dysfunctional' in relation to family life. He believes that much of what went on in child rearing in former generations was influenced heavily by the necessities of physical survival, and he calls these Stage One Cultures. In terms of child development, there was little or no attention given to the emotional needs of the child; nor were the higher goals of emotional maturity and spiritual growth given any real value. John B. Keane's play The Field (and the film based thereon) provides lucid insight into this phenomenon. The main character, 'The Bull' McCabe, hasn't spoken to his wife for fifteen years, since the suicide of their eldest son; and yet in terms of the survival ethic, this is a good match. She is a dedicated wife, who cooks, cleans and keeps the home. He for his part works hard and gives all his productive and creative energy to the field, which in turn will be passed on to the next generation. The money he saved would have provided a dowry for any daughter he might have had, which would ensure that she would find a reasonably able man who would in turn provide for her and any children. In the play however, he has no daughter and has no idea how to communicate with his other son, who is seriously emotionally damaged. Bull has no insight into this problem, but one can feel the absolute anguish growing within him as he sees that his son has no interest in the land and will take to the road with the gypsy girl.

In the Stage One societies the primary focus of the family is on creating a viable future, where the new generation can have the material necessities to survive. Little or no attention is given to communication, feelings, happiness, personal growth or any of the ethics that drive the present culture. Equally, the whole dynamic reflected in this play and in survival oriented cultures generally is seriously deficient in terms of human development, where expectations to live, create, experience joy and a certain freedom - as distinct from simply surviving and reproducing - are the main focus. Farrell argues, therefore, for the rejection of the word 'dysfunctional,' because the Stage One family was actually quite functional in terms of survival. I prefer to hold on to the label, because despite the survivor orientation of such cultures, the behaviour and treatment of children was, in my view, seriously damaging to them even in simple terms of physical and mental survival.

It is a more complex task to describe the constitution of a dysfunctional family. This is because many of its characteristics are matters of extreme behaviours. Certain dysfunctional patterns have opposite extremes, which are also dysfunctional. Several such polarised patterns are now recognised. These are: 1. Parental Conflict versus Parental Withdrawal; 2. Chaos versus Extreme Regulation; and 3. Authoritarianism versus License. Other characteristics stand alone and can be generally grouped under the heading of compulsive parental behaviour. These include: religiosity, addictions, co-dependency, violence, manipulation, inconsistency and abuse (sexual, emotional and/or physical). Each of these areas is a complex web of emotional and behavioural elements, and my descriptions will, of necessity, somewhat oversimplify the matter. Let us examine each in turn.

Parental Conflict versus Parental Withdrawal

Conflict is part of life. All partners find themselves at times in opposition to each other. In dysfunctional families, however, the conflict is ongoing and is not resolved. Continual arguing, often escalating into abusive shouting matches and even physical abuse, creates an atmosphere of fear and tension between the partners and among the children who witness it. Often, as the relationship continues to deteriorate, an uneasy truce is called and the unresolved conflicts are sent under ground. This leads to parental withdrawal. Neither parent is content or happy with the other, but has withdrawn into cold silence and superficial courtesy. This uneasy peace is frequently considered by the parents to be better for the family, especially when they choose to stay in the relationship for the sake of the children. Neither option is healthy, and children are damaged emotionally in either case.

Chaos versus Extreme Regulation

Both of these conditions are a result of parents who are out of control. The first is the direct reflection and more easily understood. The second occurs because the parents try to suppress the growing sense of chaos by applying rigorous constraints on the people within the family. In chaotic families, there is no pattern that can be relied upon to last, except the pattern that everything changes unpredictably and for no apparent reason. The family lunges from one crisis to the next. All the normally required elements for people to live together in some harmonious way are missing. Children and parents get to bed too late at night and get up too late in the morning. Getting the children ready for school is a panic-stricken frenzy, usually accompanied by hysterical shouting and running around. Financial crises abound. There is no money put aside for school books and other expenses, often leading to despair and stress that the children pick up and become worried about. Clean clothes appear irregularly, meals - when they are prepared - are of the junk food variety, children could be missing for hours without anyone noticing and the home is almost always in disarray. These families are often a reflection of immature parents: people who themselves are quite lost and don't know where they are going. This is particularly true of those who start families before they are barely out of their own adolescence.

Extreme regulation occurs among parents who have closed their minds and short-circuited their own maturing process. Such parents often have some inbred and idealistic notions about bringing up 'proper' children. These ideas are usually taken at face value from some source, such as very conservative attitudes in their own family background, rather than as an outcome of personally developed wisdom. Having closed down their own development, they are unable to cope with the exciting and unpredictable nature of young life in its formation. Extreme regulation is found in homes that are child proof, such as those with lovely white carpets in rooms where children sit on their hands and say 'excuse me', 'please may I' and 'thank you' like robots. Boredom and lack of spontaneity are hall marks of these families. Children are dressed well, but woe betide those who get their clothes dirty. Obsessive cleaning and dusting are given priority over play and recreation. Religious observances may also be considered terribly important, even when the children haven't a clue what they mean. Parental roles are rigid and unchanging and often reflect the old patriarchal model of the providing father served willingly by his courteous, but asexual, spouse. There is a kind of emotional disinfectant at work in the relationships between family members that ensures neither conflict nor creativity, neither passion nor pathos.

Authoritarianism versus License

Authoritarianism is the abuse of authority. It demands blind obedience and complete submission. It is also often accompanied by extreme regulation, which is discussed above. This form of parental control was more prevalent into the 60s and 70s. But remains prevalent in some of the more religious fundamentalist traditions. It is rooted in ideological views of the world (both religious and non-religious) where unquestioning obedience is considered to have the highest value. On a societal level, the role of blind obedience has shown devastating results. The examples of Nazi Germany, Stalin's Russia and the Cambodian massacre are all cases in point where authoritarian regimes flourished. Authoritarianism, however, can also be a family affair.

Children who grow up in such families become prepared to more easily accept being ruled by demagogues and learn to shift responsibility for their behaviour on to the shoulders of those in authority. All kinds of depraved behaviour can then be justified with the excuse 'I did it because I was obeying orders.' Living within a family run on authoritarian principles can have the effect of completely stifling the child's development of a sense of their own identity. The formation of a personality requires the process of experimentation. This process by its nature involves trying out new ideas, having unusual attitudes to things, developing one's own taste in food, music, clothes, recreational activities and so on. Authoritarianism seals off the child's desire to try new experiences and presents him with a static formula that must be accepted in order to avoid very painful consequences. A recent memoir by Tara Westover entitled Educated is a lovely read and captures the experience of growing up in a Mormon fundamentalist environment and how she managed to break free.

The other extreme of authoritarianism is that of license. This occurs when parents fail to provide healthy boundaries around certain activities in the best interest of the child. To some extent, this total freedom is a reaction to the extreme control that has reflected family values in the past. It can also be due to an effort by parents to compensate for their failure to provide adequately for the needs of their children. This is a growing concern, especially where parents are caught up in a materialistic drive to accumulate wealth, which may necessitate spending little quality time with their children. In order to assuage guilt feelings, some parents try to buy their children's loyalty and happiness by giving in to their every whim. Constant exposure to social media, TV channels and computer games come to replace relationships, and children are often given the latest gadgets to keep them occupied and out of their parents' way. Its result is the growing wave of mental health issues among young people, high levels of depression and anxiety. Juvenile crime, drug abuse and hopelessness have increased among young people of the middle-class, suburban ethos. These children, once seen as the best educated, the most articulate and well provided for, are now showing the same kinds of reactions as their more impoverished peer group, those who live and grow up in the inner cities and ghettos.

A very specific outcome of the more recent tendency to indulge children is that they often face into young adulthood with little or no resilience or capacity to cope with adversity. Psychologist Jonathan Haidt in his bestselling work "The Coddling of the American Mind" is an excellent source with regard to this growing problem. Additionally, Twenge and Campbell's "The Narcissism Epidemic" is also an important contribution that serves to warn that indulging children can lead to a huge growth in narcissistic behaviour that in turn can have seriously destructive effect on their adult lives.

Compulsive Behaviours

Many dysfunctional families are characterised by certain behaviours that in themselves are quite useful and can be healthy, but which become distorted and habitually used out of context. These are called compulsive behaviours, because the individuals lose sight of the meaning of what they are doing and become caught up in habit patterns regardless of whether the behaviour is appropriate or not. There are many such types of behaviour. Here I will deal with those that are most common and most damaging.

Religiosity

All good things can be used badly. In general, the religious ethos of most cultures is regarded as the guardian of its moral values and ethics. Religion can, however, become a force for great destruction. In many dysfunctional families, there is a type of religiosity practiced that has little to do with the great ethical statements of its teachings. It can be used instead as a method of rigid control, the suppression of life, a vehicle for prejudice and the harbinger of self-destructive guilt and shame. This form of religiosity has nothing to do with true spirituality (which will be discussed in a later section), nor the belief system that promotes love, value and respect. This religiosity is an aberration of the existing religious beliefs and used by dysfunctional parents as a weapon for control over their children.

Each major denomination has its own version. The key aspects of destructive religiosity are a denial of feelings, a belief that authority is more important than relationship, and a rigorous application of doctrinal law with no reference to its relevance to a particular situation. These situations occur when certain adults have not reached a level of moral maturity (as described by developmental psychologist Lawrence Kohlberg) to be able to distinguish the differences between the lesser of two evils and the greater of two goods. A parent, for example, can become obsessed with the rules rather than the broader moral reality that these rules try to express. He will thus always try to consign a behaviour into the categories of good and evil, rather than realise that very little in life is that simple. An example might help to illustrate this point. Let us imagine that a child lies in order to protect a friend. Here we have the juxtaposition of two rules. One, don't tell lies, and two, look after your friends. The dysfunctional person cannot cope with this complexity and will punish the lie without any reference to the motivation behind it, which is intrinsically good.

The second element of dysfunctional religious training is an emphasis on the external presentation rather than the internal workings of the heart (which is, as far as I know, the central value of all developed religion). Consequently, children are exposed to hypocrisy carried out in the name of God, which suggests to them that perhaps God is a hypocrite too.

Family rosaries were a sine qua non of the Irish family unity up to the 1960s. I have seen dozens of people who describe this practice within their family of origin while the family was being torn apart by abuse. A different, but similar, trend is discovered among many biblically based religions which justified severe physical abuse, the neglect of education, and the presence of gross material greed, all in the name of a God who is supposed to love us.

Perhaps the best analysis of this capacity for adults to justify themselves while abusing their children is found in the writings of Alice Miller, whose coinage of the term 'poisonous pedagogy' has become the benchmark for discussions in this area. In her book For Your Own Good, she gives comprehensive support - from the literature on parental guidance of the last two centuries - to her argument that religion has often been called on to justify great cruelty to children. This is still going on. One of the foremost writers on child 'psychology' within the fundamentalist New Right movement in the United States is James Dobson. In his book Dare to Discipline, first published in 1971 and in several reprints since, he writes:

... the parent's relationship with his child should be modelled after God's relationship with man 'foolishness is bound in the heart of a child; but the rod of correction shall drive it far from him', Proverbs 22:15. This recommendation has troubled some people, leading them to claim that the 'rod' was not a paddle, but a measuring stick with which to evaluate the child. The following passage was included expressly for those who were confused on that point. 'Withhold not correction from

the child; for if thou beatest him with the rod, he shall not die. Thou shalt beat him with the rod, and shalt deliver his soul from hell.' Proverbs 23:13,14. Certainly, if the 'rod' is a measuring stick, you know now what to do with it!

Having experienced such parental expressions of the love of God, it is small wonder that many young people fall prey to cults and sects who promise 'new wine for old wineskins', and who once 'converted' become again victims of abuse through religion (a thoughtful analysis of this phenomena is presented by R. A. Gilbert in his book Casting the First Stone: The Hypocrisy of Religious Fundamentalism and its Threat to Society). Similarly, so many people exposed to the 'poisonous pedagogy' reject the religion of their youth, only to return to its destructive mediocrity when they become parents themselves. They do this because they have never addressed the effects of their exposure to it on their personality development and on their ways of understanding the world. Louis Theroux's BBC documentary "The Most Hated Family in America" provide one of the most effective looks inside this type of family dysfunction. Well worth a watch to see how three generations of one family can be corrupted in the name of holiness.

Addictions

The presence of addiction within a family is now recognised as one of the most destructive of all forces. Religiosity, as discussed above, is sometimes considered such an addiction. Here, however, I will limit the discussion to those addictions that are widely recognised as such. The elements of these parental states are present in other addictions which are outside the focus of the present discussion. The primary addictions of the modern western world are addiction to mood altering substances, to work, to food, and to distraction. Much of what I have said in my book on alcoholism and the family (Children Under the Influence) is relevant and I will not repeat its contents here.

A key element in all addiction is the desire to escape from responsibility and/or suffering on the one hand, or in order to produce pleasant euphoric feelings on the other. That most addictions in themselves add new burdens to the individual and those close to him does not in itself appear to be sufficient motivation to stop the addictive process. This is due to the entrapment nature of addictive behaviour. The internal pain of the initial dysfunction is temporarily relieved by the addict through his involvement with the addictive substance, or activity. This relief sets up a vicious self-destructive cycle of pain, addictive behaviour, temporary relief, more pain, more addictive behaviour, temporary relief and so on, down a spiral of deeper and deeper despair. Robin Norwood summarises this process when she says: 'Addiction develops when reliance on the drug, substance or activity evolves from being a choice into being a compulsion.'

The abuse of tolerance building chemicals, including alcohol, illegal drugs and prescription medications, shows this cycle most clearly because of the nature of these substances. Addiction to one's own bodily chemicals through the adrenaline surges involved in excessive exercise, gambling, outbursts of aggression and other activities that do not require ingesting a substance is just as destructive, but not as obvious, to the onlooker.

When people become caught in the trap of addiction their ability to provide any form of stable or healthy environment for the family is seriously undermined. Gradually, the whole family becomes caught up with the addict's turmoil. Some try to save him or her and waste huge emotional resources in the process. Others become victims of the addict's acting out, being verbally and sometimes physically violated, especially where substance abuse is concerned. Still others lose the financial resources required to provide even the basic necessities. The workaholic family is often well provided for in material terms, but the atmosphere is suffused with stress when the workaholic is present; or conversely, the family members are neglected through long absences. Families where there is parental addiction cannot function in a way that promotes the healthy development of the people in it.

Co-dependency

Alongside 'dysfunctional' the word 'co-dependency' is in vogue in describing one of the major unhealthy parental patterns in dysfunctional families. I will discuss this problem at length in a further chapter, because it is one of the outcomes of growing up in a dysfunctional home. Here I wish to describe briefly the effect of parental co-dependency on the family unit.

Co-dependency is a personality disorder, which has at its root the failure of a person to develop an identity and singularity that is not dependent on something or somebody else. It is most clearly seen in relationships where a person tries to live his or her life through another person. Because it is a disordered condition, the relationship is almost always with another disordered person. Rarely will a healthy individual with an intact sense of identity want to stay in a relationship with a co-dependent person. Rather, co dependents are attracted to people whose identity is in some way fragmented. The formula for relationships that has often been encouraged is one which says that two incomplete people marry or become partners to make a unit of one (often as a result of misinterpreting the religious teaching that the 'two shall become as one'). This is the formula for a co-dependent relationship which can have devastating results for the people involved.

In a family which is headed by such a relationship there is a great deal of emotional entanglement and enmeshing. Neither parent has an intact identity. They look to each other to provide what their parents didn't provide for them. This leads to a long, fruitless and frustrating search, which ends up in unhappiness and lack of fulfilment. This is often experienced in the sexual arena, where the boundaries between the unfulfilled affection and tenderness needs of the child within the adult become confused with adult sexual needs. As a consequence, many co-dependent couples have sexual difficulties. Children who grow up in families where co-dependency is a problem (a significant number I suspect) are at best exposed to unhealthy models of relationships; and at worst become entangled in the emotional web, thus becoming emotionally damaged and co-dependent themselves.

Violence

One of the most dramatic forms of family dysfunction is that of violence. It is also perhaps the most obviously destructive. When violence within a family refers to intense and forceful physical attack, usually as a result of a breakdown of emotional control. There are some people, however, who can be calculatedly violent, which suggests even greater levels of emotional sickness. Violence strikes at the heart of a person's dignity, because it violates all the dimensions of his being. It causes physical pain, emotional trauma and cognitive distortion all at the same time. Violence also breeds violence. It is ironic that many people who have been influenced by religious teachings that encourage physically beating their children forget the wise saying that 'he who lives by the sword shall die by the sword'. Violence between partners is almost always accompanied by violence towards children. The partner who beats his wife will rarely control that tendency when dealing with the children. Similarly, the victim of spousal abuse will sometimes take out their rage against the children. And again, many children who experience physical violence growing up will, as adults, visit such violence on their own families. It is more difficult for them to try to reach an understanding of a child's behaviour, to seek its hidden meaning and to solve problems creatively and helpfully. As a consequence, physical violence is always an easy trend into which they can slip. I sometimes wonder how an adult who beats his or her children would feel if someone treated them that way when they make a mistake, or do something that is unpopular or against 'the rules'. Children who are violated by their parents or witness such violation between partners are deeply scarred by the experience. I will discuss these effects in more detail in a later section.

Manipulation

Manipulation is a common characteristic of dysfunctional families. The children and adults in the family are manipulated into roles that become rigid and unchanging. Each role is required so that the emotional dynamics of the family can continue to run smoothly, even though these dynamics are destructive to all the family members. When someone tries to break the mould by resisting the role in which he or she is functioning, the family rally around to try to make that person continue in their expected position. Some examples may help to clarify this point. Let us take the situation of a family where there is an addicted parent. Usually some member of the family will take the role of the hero. This child has the responsibility of giving dignity to the family unit usually through being over-responsible, achieving highly in school and other activities, and not showing his vulnerability.

Eventually the child comes to be seen in that role alone, and his vulnerability or need to stop being so responsible and hardworking is no longer tolerated. The other family members need to have someone like this in the family and will react negatively should this person stop functioning in this way. Similarly, one of the children will most likely become the emotional caretaker. This is the child who will offer the others emotional support and sustenance, regardless of his own needs and hurts. The other children, and in some cases the co-dependent spouse, will rely on this child emotionally. If this child cannot or will not continue in this role, then he will experience hostility and rejection from the others. This will obviously hurt a child with such sensitivity, and the likelihood is that he will return to what is familiar and try to get his own needs met through caring for others. In this scenario, we see a child being manipulated into a role that is destructive to his development, and central to this kind of manipulation is the problem of conditional love.

Conditional love occurs when each family member is given love, attention or affirmation only as a response to fulfilling the emotional needs of the family. Because the family is dysfunctional, many of these needs are inappropriate, such as those expressed when a child has to become a parent to his parents or to his/her siblings. Dysfunctional families are unable to provide unconditional love, because none of the family members are integrated and mature enough to provide for others in this way. Conditional love is by its nature manipulative. Once manipulation grows out of conditional love, the die is cast for children to service the needs of the family through taking on roles that are eventually destructive to their development and which produce serious problems in adult life. Strongly related to manipulation is parental immaturity. When parents are emotionally immature and often troubled, the result is that there are unpredictable mood swings and often wild changes of behaviour. The parents are not sufficiently developed in themselves to act in a consistent, healthy manner. Children who, by their nature, want to love and model after the parents are given a myriad of different and sometimes contradictory messages about what is expected of them. This results in confusion and insecurity. Children who grow up with such inconsistency develop problems in relation to having a clear sense of their own identity. It's as if they internalize the inconsistency of their parents and become confused about themselves.

Abuse

Abuse within a family can be categorized as physical, sexual and/ or emotional. Any of these grow out of a combination of two factors.

The first is the presence of an emotionally impaired or immature parent. The second is the enduring myth that parents own their children, and that they can therefore treat them badly and act out their immaturity or emotional sickness on them. I will briefly describe the features of each kind of abuse.

I have already discussed the problem of violence within the family. Such violence is only one form of physical abuse. It is generally characterised by the parent lashing out in a rage and usually has no belief system about what is good for children underlying it. There is a broader aspect to physical abuse, which usually includes some element of justification for hurting children physically in terms of it being good for their development. A great deal of destruction to the growing child can result from physical abuse used under the guise of responsible parenting. In general, physical abuse consists of hitting, punching pinching, dragging children by the hair or ears, and other forms of hurting children physically. The parent can be of the opinion that this is necessary in order for children to learn respect and obedience. It is ironic the number of parents who think that they can teach a child respect whilst showing no respect for them. Respect by its nature is not something that can be enforced. It is an attitude of mind that grows when children see parents respecting themselves and acting respectfully towards others.

Sexual abuse consists of three levels, The first level is sometimes a result of parental ignorance rather than a conscious desire to use the child for the parent's gratification (a key element in all sexual abuse). This area can include insensitivity to the child's bodily integrity; not allowing sufficient privacy; allowing him to see sexual activity either between the parents or on television (that is inappropriate to his/her age) The second level is based on verbal and visual signals that are sexual in content and from which an adult gains sexual gratification: talking about sex or sexual organs in a way that titillates the parent's sexual appetite; exposing oneself in a sexual way; or looking at the child while undressing in a sexually oriented way. This is second level abuse, which the child picks up and internalises, resulting in a game of sexual flirtation or enormous self-consciousness and shame; these in turn can have devastating effects on the child's sexuality in later life. The third level of abuse is actual physical molestation, which ranges from various forms of stroking and touching in a sexual way to full anal or vaginal penetration. This latter area is often misunderstood by people as the only form of sexual abuse. This is mainly because it is a grosser form of abuse, is criminalised by society and draws the attention of the media. Sexual abuse, even in its milder forms, can have life-shattering consequences. To some degree, the damaging consequences of sexual abuse are mediated by the nature of the abuse, the temperament of the child and the resources available to the child in being able to tell someone and receive care and attention in response to the experience.

Three areas are particularly relevant in understanding how such abuse damages children. It is firstly an invasion of the child at his or her most tender years which can cause havoc with his or her emotional, physical and intellectual formation. This results in a breakdown in the child's ability to develop a healthy sense of him- or herself, and a secure identity.

Secondly, it is a grave betrayal of the child by the adult world. This is particularly true when the abuser is a family member or trusted adult (this is most often the case). The child then develops a no-trust rule, which can lead to withdrawal and isolation. Sexual violation may also leave the person living in a degree of fear, which can range from chronic low-level anxiety to extreme terror.

Thirdly, it damages the child's sexual development. This has the result of producing a wide variety of sexual problems in adulthood. All of these areas of damage will usually become apparent in later life, even when the memories of the abuse are no longer in conscious awareness (for a useful and more in-depth analysis of this area, see Gay Search's book The Last Taboo, Sexual Abuse of Children).

All forms of abuse include a dimension of emotional violation, but emotional abuse can occur on its own, separate from the other areas discussed above. This type of abuse is reflected in verbal assault, where children are screamed at regularly, or conversely given cold, unforgiving and silent treatment. Emotional abuse is the conscious effort of the adult to hurt the child's feelings, to cause them inner pain and to turn him against himself. This latter aspect is important, because children will almost always blame themselves for the emotional state of their parents. This is doubly true when the parent actively blames the child for his or her own feelings. Other forms of emotional abuse occur when parents unfavourably compare children to others inside or outside the family, when they tease them about their weaknesses, or ridicule them in any way.

Emotional abuse is the favoured weapon of parents who are passively hostile. They can express their hostility indirectly, which causes the child to become very confused. They experience the pain of teasing and ridicule, but are left wondering whether they should be hurt by what is being said. Emotional abuse is therefore very insidious. It works like a poison inside the developing child, leaving traces of emotional pain and heartbreak within.

Summary

A dysfunctional family is one which reflects any one of the above characteristics as an intrinsic and ongoing part of the operation of the family. There is, thus, a wide range of dysfunctionality, from its milder form where there may be intermittent experiences of one of the less devastating characteristics, to the grossly disturbed families where several of the above descriptions are a regular feature of the family relationships. In the next section I will examine the results of growing up in such families.

Thus far I have discussed the family in some detail. This is because it is a child's experiences within the family unit during the formative years that have most lasting consequences. Many very worthwhile books deal primarily with the family as the place wherein children are damaged. I am thinking particularly of John Bradshaw's book Bradshaw on the Family and Charles Whitfield's Healing the Child Within. These and others present excellent material on the subject. Alongside the experiences within the family, there are other significant areas of influence that can also have long-term effects, for good or ill, on a child. After the family influences, the experiences within school are next in importance. It is to this issue we now turn.

CHAPTER 4
The Experience of School

Introduction

Most children spend a large amount of their crucial developmental years at school. During those years, they are exposed to three aspects of life: a social peer group; an authority system; and an enforced set of learning tasks. All of these are considered by educators to be important vehicles for preparing children for adult life. This preparation can have a lasting influence on how the person adjusts to living in the adult world. Some of these influences can be very constructive, whilst others can be very damaging. School experience is a two-edged sword. This is particularly so when a child is growing up in a dysfunctional family. Many opportunities arise whereby the unhealthy influences of the home can either be relieved or exacerbated through the child's involvement in school.

Some commentators believe that the whole institutional aspect of taking children away from parents to educate them in large groups is, in itself, damaging. I have some sympathy with this view. More specifically, our notions of education and learning have been strongly influenced by the industrial revolution, and still reflect certain elements of that historical epoch. In particular, the industrial revolution has led to the rigorous structuring of adult life and the artificial division of work and recreation. In order to prepare children for their place in industrialised society, school gives them early experiences of having their time structured from the outside and regulated by the bell. As a result, they are more amenable to the adult world of work, despite its often discussed alienation and meaninglessness. This could cynically be described as training little rats for the big rat race. Similarly, the artificial division which separates learning from play is also a training ground for other experiences later in life, the most important of these being the separation of leisure from work and the creative process from the productive process in the adult world of work.

Now that we live in the post-industrialised era, that of information technology and robotics, it will be interesting to see the effects of these formative educational experiences. Will they have produced the very characteristics in our young adults that make them unable to adjust to a post-industrial society? Will increased leisure time, greater need for creativity, adaptability and abstract thinking present serious problems for young adults in trying to adjust to a world for which they are ill-prepared? Some believe that this has already happened. One of the most eloquent contributors to this phenomenon is Harari (2016) who suggests that modern information technology is converting human beings into data, to be interpreted and influenced through the development of computer algorithms. He writes:

In this, humans are similar to other domesticated animals. We have bred docile cows that produce enormous amounts of milk, but are otherwise far inferior to their wild ancestors. They are less agile, less curious and resourceful. We are now creating tame humans that produce enormous amounts of data and function as very efficient chips in a huge data-processing mechanism, but these data cows hardly maximise the human potential. Indeed we have no idea what the full potential is....If we are not careful, we will end up with downgraded humans misusing upgraded computers to wreak havoc on themselves and the world. (p 71)

These issues are of grave importance, and reflect deep philosophical questions relating to the role and practice of education in our modern world. They are, however, only peripheral to the task of this book. I merely wish to suggest that, although I will be discussing certain aspects of schooling in terms of its effects on children, there are broader questions regarding the phenomenon of schooling itself which require attention.

In general, there are two categories of school environment. Firstly, there is the environment that provides the kind of understanding and treatment of children that gives them what they need in order to emerge from childhood well equipped educationally and socially to take a creative and productive place in today's world. Secondly, there is the environment that creates such problems for children that their personalities, self-esteem and ability to learn become damaged. Again, it is useful to categorise these school environments as healthy or dysfunctional, respectively.

Healthy School Environment

There are three main elements in a healthy educational environment: 1. the teacher's attitudes and abilities; 2. the relevance of the curriculum; and 3. the social organisation of the school. I will not deal with these in detail. My purpose here is to provide a context in which dysfunctional schooling can be understood more clearly.

The Teacher's Attitudes and Abilities

The teacher's role in the school environment is central. His or her attitudes to children and his or her ability to work well with them provide the cornerstone of modern education. The teacher is also a significant role model for the children in his or her care. Teaching is a vocation. As such, it requires a commitment from the whole person. One cannot function well as a teacher and treat it just like any other job. I believe the key attitudes in being the kind of teacher who promotes healthy learning among children are: a liking for children; a flexible and adaptable approach; sensitivity; and emotional stability. These characteristics cannot be taught in training school, but yet are the foundation on which teaching skills can be built. Teachers who do not reflect these attributes generally become very stressed and unhappy in their work. This in turn often leads to conflict in the classroom, which turns the children away from the teacher and creates greater turmoil and unhappiness for all concerned. I recently read the memoir "Poor" by Katriona

O'Sullivan. It is a wonderful story of resilience and courage as she battled to survive against the odds of a terrible traumatic childhood. One of the most beautiful passages is her description of a teacher who, seeing the terrible conditions she lived in, sensitively and carefully helped her.

The key abilities that teachers who promote healthy development in children possess are, in my opinion, as follows: excellent social skills; an ability to communicate clearly to those intellectually less developed; a good knowledge of the subjects being taught; and an interest in further learning. This latter point, in particular, is rarely given enough emphasis. It seems ironic that while school is considered to be the place where a hunger for learning is considered central, the teachers' own attitudes in this regard are given little consideration. Desire is a human emotion, and a desire to learn is better caught than taught. Small wonder, then, that many children reflect a lack of interest in learning when they sit for hours every day in the presence of an adult who communicates (often unconsciously) boredom with the job. These attitudes and abilities, while central to a healthy experience of school, are only one aspect of the totality of children's experience within the school environment.

The Relevance of the Curriculum

The curriculum of any educational establishment is the stated content of what is to be taught. I do not wish to involve myself in a comprehensive discussion of the complex aspects of curriculum development. It is true, however, that what children learn or don't learn in school has a dramatic influence on their lives. The relevance of a curriculum refers to whether or not what a child learns has any bearing on what his or her life as an adult will require from him or her.

In my view, there are four elements in a relevant curriculum. These are the degree to which the learning tasks of school help or hinder the child in becoming someone who is able to: learn to think through and solve problems; have the ability to develop new skills; achieve mastery in a set of skills (such as reading and writing); and keep a set of information stored in the memory which can be called upon when required. We can see, therefore, that learning in school involves developing the ability to continue learning in adulthood, and not just acquiring a basic set of information and skills. Much education up to recent times has emphasised the latter, leading many people to spend years in school without learning anything remotely related to where they find themselves in adult life. Indeed, it could also be said that much of the curriculum formation resulted in people being unable to think for themselves, an ironic outcome of what is called education. In this context, the now iconic work of Paolo Freire (2017), even if somewhat dated, remains a source of deep insight. His juxtaposing what he terms the "'narration sickness'" of contemporary education with that of dialogical learning has much to offer. In the former he tells us that:

"Narration (with the teacher as narrator) leads the students to memorise the narrated content. Worse still it turns them into containers, into receptacles to be filled by the teacher. The more completely he fills the receptacle, the better a teacher he is. The more meekly the receptacles permit themselves to be filled, the better the students they are."

It is important to qualify this critique with the observation that there are certain realms of knowledge where a narration approach is not only valuable but is essential to learning. There are subject areas that require factual empirical grounding. It would be absurd to try to learn trigonometry, organic chemistry, or pilot training by having animated discussions and opinion sharing about them! We are also witnessing now the entry of ideological training in young children's classes, which to my mind is deeply concerning, We have only just left the scene where young children were indoctrinated with religious propaganda only to find now some new ideologies, more specifically, gender identity theory is being introduced. I fear this will do more harm than good in the longer term.

The Social Organisation of the School

Both the quality of the teaching and the relevance of the learning tasks occur in a social climate within the school. It is in this social context that many beliefs about how people should relate to each other evolve. More specifically, the social organisation of a school comprises its efforts to promote healthy social interaction between pupils and teachers and amongst each other. A healthy social environment is one where children learn the importance of relationships and the skills to communicate effectively. Several dimensions of this area are worth discussion. In a healthy school environment, relationships among the staff are respectful and courteous. Teachers respect and value the pupils. There is no humiliation, abuse or isolation of pupils. Pupils are expected to treat their teachers with the same kind of respect that they are given. Young people are not allowed to bully, intimidate, mock or hurt others. Conflict between the staff is kept away from the watchful eyes of the pupils. The whole school acts as a team, with the common goal of encouraging a hunger for learning as well as imparting skills and knowledge.

This description of a healthy learning environment may appear, at least until more recent times, idealistic and utopian. The description of dysfunctional schooling was, over the last century of formal education, a far more familiar scenario. It is to this that we now turn.

Dysfunctional Schooling

This book focuses on healing the hurts of childhood. As such, it is important to stress the fact that not all the damage to children comes about within their families. Dysfunctional schooling can result in grave emotional damage to children. This area of experience in a child's life has improved dramatically in the past three decade, so much of what follows here is not so relevant to readers who did not have to endure the kinds of cruelty often meted out to those in earlier years. For those of us educated before the 1970s, there is a legacy of damage to be confronted and dealt with. This legacy comprises the following, characteristics of education for most of the last two centuries: 1. Mistreatment by teachers; 2. Bullying; 3. Preferential treatment based on ability and social class; 4. The cultivation of inferiority among those less gifted. All of these have been characteristic, to a greater or lesser extent, of the schooling received by a majority of people who are now over fifty years old. Those children who came from secure and healthy homes, while damaged to some extent by exposure to these influences, were less harmed than those who had no secure foundation to begin with. And ironically, it is these other, more vulnerable, children who were most likely to suffer greater torment within the hallowed halls of academe. Like many areas in life, the already weak were treated with most disdain.

Mistreatment by Teachers

Here's a story from my own experience at the age of 10. Martin (not his real name) was ten years old and unable to protect himself from the worst excesses of a violent and cruel teacher Those who were at the top of the class were saved from the worst ravages of this man, although most did not escape. Martin, however, was the one who suffered most. He was obviously a distressed child. His clothes were unkempt and dirty, his hair unwashed and his body hunched slightly in the vigilance and fear that characterises those who are afraid of life. His face had an expression of loneliness and despair and his forehead furrowed in a permanent frown. Whoever his parents were, they did not care for him. This much was obvious to those willing to see the obvious. He was always late for school.

Who can guess the turmoil out of which he came each day to that dreaded place of learning called school? His classmates sat, frightened and tense, not knowing where the axe would fall. And, selfishly, like most children, they were relieved in knowing that Martin's late arrival would temporarily take the focus off them. And so it did. Each day he arrived late, after the work of the day had begun, sometimes by up to half an hour. His friends would watch the handle of the door turn slowly and wonder how this young boy, their own age, must feel, heading once again into the maw of the teacher's cruelty.

Evil has an inherent fascination. So the other pupils watched, their tender young minds perverted by the scene of cruelty as this supposedly responsible adult beat Martin with a cane as hard as he could. Martin's response was always the same: his colour flowered up along his neck and face as the pain and humiliation registered through his young efforts to keep from crying out, and to hold on to whatever threads of dignity remained in his already damaged soul.

I don't know where he is now. Maybe he has found some peace. Martin's experience is instructive, because it was a hallmark of school experience for some who were educated in Ireland up to the 1970's. This was particularly the case for boys. The savagery of some teachers was reserved for boys, the taboo of physical cruelty to girls holding in check the worst excesses of certain teachers' aggression. The female version of this kind of cruelty married a milder form of physical abuse with a more insidious form of psychological torment. That these happenings were tolerated by other more caring teachers, and by a large number of parents, and by the Catholic church whose mandate was to treat children with dignity care and compassion. is a grave indictment on the society of that time

Bullying

In earlier times it is not surprising that bullying, which can have a devastating effect on a child, was a regular occurrence within schools of that period. I have already alluded to the perversion of young minds by having been exposed to adult role models who were bullies, it is only a short step to partake in beating and humiliating those weaker than oneself. Many children of that period lived in fear from the violence of those stronger than them within the school environment. Certain children who themselves were beaten at home, and beaten again in school, displaced all the pent-up rage on their peers.

In girls' schools, bullying often reflected the emotional abuse experienced at the hands of some teachers. Young girls were tormented emotionally, marginalised from their peer groups, mocked and laughed at. And again, it was often those most vulnerable and unable to cope who were singled out for this treatment. Mistreatment by teachers is no longer a feature of modern-day education. However, the phenomenon of bullying remains a serious challenge. In its more modern form the use of social media to marginalize and mistreat individuals selected out for such treatment can lead to very serious emotional distress and is often a feature of suicidal thoughts and sometimes action. Psychologist Steven Hassan explains that the great hope that social media platforms would improve interpersonal relationships is premature. He writes that *"The nature of so many comments on social media seems to indicate otherwise. Nastiness, Schadenfreude, and dismissive characterizations of opposing opinions substitute for dialogue. Internet platforms are structured to get a payout from high emotion and clickability. Canceling and calling-out posts fit perfectly into that paradigm. Commenting is instantly rewarding, and nasty and demeaning comments .... allow commenters to feel morally and intellectually superior.". Often these effects on a young person are kept hidden from the family until it is too late*

Preferential Treatment

Two aspects of the pupils' life seem to have been particularly susceptible to preferential treatment: social status and intellectual ability. Those who came from the 'right side of town' were more likely to avoid the abuse and taunting of the more disturbed teachers. It was easier to get away with hurting a child who was already impoverished than one whose parents held a prestigious place in society. It is likely that such parents would not feel intellectually or socially inferior to the teacher, who was also in many cases a clergyman or a nun. Parents whose roots lay in the poorer and less respected classes had, to a large extent, been brought up with a feel ng of inferiority. These people would he less likely to challenge authority or question the behaviour of their social superiors.

Similarly, within the class environment those who were more naturally equipped to deal with the abstraction of academic work were treated with more respect and value than others less able. Conversely, those given special treatment in class were more likely to be mistreated by their peers, because they could perceive the unfairness of what was happening in terms of the teacher's reactions. They took out their hurt on the more intellectually gifted, and often resorted to the bullying referred to above.

A similar, but even more destructive, phenomenon occurred regularly when children were set apart for special abuse by certain teachers. These were the opposite of the teacher's pet——the teacher's scapegoat. Most classes had one or two fulfilling the role. These were often children who were generally intellectually weak and emotionally vulnerable. They became the scapegoats who were offered up by the class as a means of providing relief from the tension, boredom and fear that often accompanied the experience of school. They were often funny and almost always in trouble. But deep down they knew that they were never going to achieve anything. The luckier ones dropped out of school early and found a place in society through apprenticeships in trades. Others had to continue in the farce of continual academic failure and live with the label of being stupid and dull.

The Cultivation of Inferiority

In every competition there are winners and losers. One of the most destructive elements of dysfunctional schooling is that it sets up learning and education as a competition. As a consequence, the focus changes from developing a love of learning for its own sake to a desperate struggle to do better than others, to get ahead, or to avoid disgrace. A young person's love of knowledge can be practically destroyed by making it a tool for success rather than an experience that is in itself worth pursuing. Central to this issue is the view that most people do not want to learn. In response to this belief, there was a need to force children, by some means or other, to learn. Two methods were commonly used: physical abuse and punishment; and shame and derision. In recent times, the use of physical torment for failing academically has disappeared, but the use of shame continues as a powerful incentive. The pain of failure remains an intense motivational force for some children within education.

Psychologists now realise that continual experiences of failure breed a hopeless, helpless view of life. Children who are consistently confronted by academic failure develop feelings of inferiority. These feelings in turn produce a greater fear of failure, often expressed as an unwillingness to try to learn. When this happens, the person then fails, and in so doing experiences more inferiority, leading again to more fear and then to giving up. One solution now being applied is I believe making things worse. This is the notion that in order to protect young people from the pain involved in realizing that others are just better at some things, its better to dumb down the system. This is going to destroy the important role of standards in education, which is of critical importance to the economic and social success of any society. Protecting people from reality even if painful is not a solution.

Any educational system that cultivates competition within education runs the risk of leaving a significant number of young people upset by the experience. This is because there is an intrinsic unfairness within this approach. Not all children have the same levels of academic prowess, and even those who are gifted can come from widely different backgrounds, some which encourage the developing child along the path of learning and others that take little interest in, or actively discourage, such activity. Then there is the issue that in the past, much academic learning was extremely narrow and emphasised certain skills at the expense of others. So the deck was stacked unfairly from the outset against those children who did not measure up to the standards being set. To value the worth of young people in their formative years on this basis is to set them up to struggle with inferiority, sometimes for the rest of their lives. To combat this requires constructing the educational system in such a way as there is room for everyone to achieve a dignified standard in areas particularly suited to their abilities.

Thankfully, the modern approach to educating children shows more enlightenment and a more holistic orientation to learning. At post-primary level, however, the race for academic success continues unabated, leaving huge numbers with a sense of futility about what should be one of the joys of life, namely curiosity to learn and the sense of achievement that comes with knowing and understanding. For many adults who read this book, their experience within school of two or three decades ago will have left numerous scars on their self-esteem and self-confidence.

Summary

This chapter has examined some of the influences of school experience on the development of children. The benefits of education are generally of real value to a developing person. Recent decades have seen the evolution of schooling into a far more beneficial period in a child's life than heretofore. It can be said, however, that until relatively recent times, the cruelty expressed toward children - either in making them direct victims of physical beatings and humiliation, or in terms of having to witness such deeds have left often life- long scars. These traumatic events, including those where psychological mistreatment was a feature, often remain unresolved and carry over into adult life. As such, these experiences need to be addressed as part of understanding oneself and healing the legacy of the past. These issues will be discussed further in a later part of the book. The third major area of influence in the formative years is that of the peer group, and it is to this issue we now turn.

CHAPTER 5
Adolescence

'When I was fourteen, I thought my father was the most ignorant man in the world, when I became eighteen, I was amazed at how much he had learned.'

Mark Twain

Gerry's parents were frantic when they telephoned me for an appointment. Their fourteen-year-old son had just been delivered home by the police. They found him so drunk that he was unable to walk. This event was just one of a series of incidences that led them to believe Gerry was in serious trouble. His school work was continuing to deteriorate, his attitude to his parents was negative, bordering on the hostile, and they were finding great difficulty in coping with his rejection of their authority. Because I believe that in many instances, parents are a child's best counsellors I suggested we meet together. During the discussion, it became clear that a major issue for the parents related to Gerry's friends, all of whom seemed, in their opinion, to be drop-outs.

Gerry sat silently as they provided me with a litany of his misdemeanours. His body language showed him to be defensive and his face carried a rather cynical smirk. His parents, on the other hand, were obviously distressed, and yet seemed to bear little anger and a good deal of concern about what was happening to their son. Realising that there was little point at this stage in trying to pry Gerry loose from his guarded approach, I asked to speak with him alone. What evolved in that discussion is something I have seen many times among young people trying to assert their individuality.

Gerry turned out to be a very bright young man in the midst of an identity crisis. He was very shrewd, and realised that his parents were unable to understand what was going on inside his active mind. He showed a great deal of insight into himself and into the problems that he encountered. Much of his difficulty centred on his struggle with accepting his mother's strong religious beliefs, and her struggle to enforce these on him. Not wanting to hurt her, and yet not believing in her views and wishing to let go of many of the religious practices, left him with little option but to withdraw from her. All of this was going on behind the facade of a cynical, uncaring teenager. It is during such times of vulnerability that young people find comfort and security with others their own age. And thus peer-group pressure begins to take over as a commanding influence in the life of a person during this formative stage.

The Peer Group

We are accustomed to thinking of peer-group pressure in relation to teenage years rather than as a facet of life that, for most of us, is an intrinsic part of living. Most people have a peer group of some sort. These are the people with whom we find most identification, such as our work colleagues, our social network, or those with whom we share some common interest, from sport to discussions of child rearing. One of the reasons why we tend to think about peer group pressure as an adolescent phenomenon is that, in general, this group becomes noticeable to the adult world because it provides a forum for young people to rebel against the status quo while still having the safety net of the group. This can be exacerbated when parents abdicate their responsibility to continue communicating and building a new type of relationship with their adolescent children.

A second reason is that, from the outside, it appears that the group is exerting strong influence on the individual to act in ways that are not acceptable to his parents, or to society in general. Common characteristics of such groups are an interest in things radical, such as rebellious and anarchic music. Clothes that are striking and sometimes considered unaesthetic, hair style and jewellery that flaunt acceptable modes of appearance - all become the uniform for young peoples' attempt to reject the conditioning and value system of society. This is a necessary part of healthy development, because the crucial stage of adolescence is a time when the individual tries to establish a sense of identity. In becoming a person in their own right, they must take an opportunity to reject the status quo, to try out new modes of being in the world, and in so doing find a value system and a way of living of their own.

The crisis of adolescence occurs when strong pressure is brought to bear on the young person to accept a ready-made formula from his family, rather than experiment with new ideas. The peer group is the forum for trying out these new ways of thinking and behaving. It can be said, however, that during this period of life the person is extremely vulnerable and can get completely lost, for they do not yet have the maturity to withstand some of the pressures that can occur. Without the security of knowing that the family - especially parents - are allies even during a time of rebellion, they can find himself adrift on the sea of life with no aids to navigate its sometimes treacherous waters. Those who have been rejected by their parents have only the guidance of the peer group which is, in itself, unsure and insecure.

The task of adolescence is the formation of identity. It is this identity that provides the young person with the map for adult life. Peer-group influence can have a powerful say in how this occurs. We will look at three outcomes that occur in this process. Two are dysfunctional, and the third is the healthy progression through adolescence.

Dysfunctional Formation of Identity

Young people do not reach their teenage years with a blank slate. In addition to an inborn set of traits and sensitivities, they have already been strongly influenced in the formation of personality by the forces for good or ill discussed above. Those who have been exposed to healthy, consistent love and a respecting, encouraging education are in a far better position to take on the challenges and trials of adolescent years than those who have been used, abused and ridiculed, in either the family or at school.

Many people arrive on the threshold of adolescence with a fairly intact sense of themselves, an optimistic outlook on life and a security in knowing that they are loved, even if not fully understood. They will be inclined to select a peer group that reflects some value and respect for the adult world, while still trying out new ideas and behaviours. They will be less likely to become destructive to themselves or others, and will tend to leave a group that operates in this way. Others come into these turbulent years with very little self-esteem, a gnawing emptiness within and a fearful and somewhat hopeless outlook on life. It is this latter group who are most likely to find adolescence extremely traumatic. In losing their way, they may become casualties to peer-group influences that set them up for a life of strife and failure. They will most likely select a peer group that reflects the anger and disappointment of their early years, and their rebellion will be far more than the natural process of questioning and experimenting. Together with other dejected and angry teenagers, they become part of a group, or gang, that will be suffused with anger and destruction. One recent example that is quite frightening has emerged with the massive growth of the online world. The phenomenon that is referred to as incels (involuntary celibates) are a group of young, and some not so young men who cultivate together a hatred of women because they are failing in their efforts to establish any successful intimate sexual relationships.

What we notice here is that adolescents tend to choose the group that operates in a way that allows their own level of emotional health, or ill health, to find expression. Adults looking on will often be tempted, as part of their own denial, to blame the peer group, rather than realise that the young person is only finding expression for what is inside him or her in the company of others who are also emotionally damaged.

Identity Diffusion

Young people in this latter group will tend to experience what is called 'identity diffusion'. This occurs as one possible out come in the formation of identity, and comprises a loss of a sense of direction and a confusion about oneself in terms of personal, career and social identity. The young person cannot locate any internal guiding principles and experiences a deep sense of doubt; he or she can be aptly as one who doubts is like the surf of the sea, driven and tossed by the wind.' The wind in this analogy is most likely to be the influence of other confused adolescents who are also lost. The internal strife that accompanies such confusion will often lead beyond experimentation with drink and drugs into dependency on these chemicals in order to ease emotional distress. Similarly, the rebellion against the status quo turns gradually into a jealous anger, as the young person observes others growing up and making their way - albeit tentatively through these years of self-conscious formation.

Identity Foreclosure

A second outcome that sometimes occurs during adolescence is that of 'identity foreclosure'. This refers to the closing down of oneself, and a refusal to navigate the swirling currents by staying at home in the safety of the port. Young people who elect this course are often too frightened of life and too suppressed by their parental and authority figures to venture into life as individuals. Rather, they select the safety of a rigid and pre-packaged way of being in the world. Choosing socially acceptable career paths that are the desire of their parents, acting like adults with their peer group and generally quashing the energy that drives them towards unique individuality, they live 'provisional lives', and may never experience the joy of becoming a person in their own right.

In my work as a counsellor, I meet many people in their thirties and forties whose lives reflect either of these out comes. The former group are still trying to find out who they are. A good number will have spent their twenties twisting and turning in a struggle to find a place for themselves. Many have difficulty and frustration in their working lives, being haunted by a sense of not being in the right place, and full of regrets about their failures in education and relationships. Those in the latter group are haunted by different demons. Having spent a decade or two in a well-ordered effort to make the 'right' choices and do the 'right' things, they are left with a sense of emptiness and mediocrity that seems to mark out their existence. This often leads them into a quiet despair of ever being able to take life into their own hands.

Identity Resolution

Midway between the extremes of identity diffusion and identity foreclosure is the healthy outcome of 'identity resolution'. Children who come into the uncharted waters of adolescence with a sense of dignity and worth, and with a deep sense of their parents' love and support, will pass through this develop mental journey with few permanent scars. The worries and self-consciousness of this time are underpinned by an optimism that things will turn out all right. The ability to talk about one's concerns with adults who at least to some extent seem to understand, and the lack of a repressive and overly strict regime bode well for the developing young adult. Questions concerning one's emerging sexuality - how to deal with sexual feelings, attraction to the opposite sex, one's body image - become exciting, if somewhat terror-stricken, adventures. Questions about one's place in the world and the universe, the meaning of existence and the purpose of life, can be asked of oneself and others with the secure knowledge that it all doesn't have to be sorted out right away. An emerging interest in a life task such as a vocation or career begin to tug at the heartstrings, seeking a way forward through education or training.

During adolescence, all these issues begin to become clearer when the youth is given the freedom to explore and find solutions within the security of a loving family. Gradually, the confusion begins to ease, as the person settles into a firm sense of themselves. The task of adult life can then begin. This is the resolution of identity, which will sustain and contain a person throughout life's crises and challenges.

Summary

This short chapter concerned itself with peer group influence during adolescence. The key point in my understanding of this process is that we tend to choose a peer group that reflects our own emotional condition and this is, to a large extent, determined by our childhood experiences within our family and later within school. I don't think it is useful to see peer group influence as completely separate from these other influences.

In general, a person integrates the experiences of adolescence into his or her sense of identity. If a lot of pain and trauma is experienced during this time, it will seriously affect the sense of identity that emerges, which in turn provides the patterns of living that are used during adulthood. It is to the issue of adulthood, and to the effects of these formative experiences in adult life, that we now turn.

Part Two
Dysfunctional Living

CHAPTER 6
The Walking Wounded

Hurt People Hurt People
Josephine Hart.

Introduction

As I reflect on beginning this chapter, I am visited by some images from the original version of the film All Quiet on the Western Front. I remember watching it as a young teenager being moved by the tenderness between the soldiers amidst the awful carnage and degradation of trench warfare. I was particularly touched by one special moment of compassion. Two soldiers, one English and one German, fought with each other in a crater, leaving one soldier dying while the other, the perpetrator of his death, began to discover, with wonder and terrible sadness, the humanity of the enemy whom he had just fatally wounded. A second image is that of two buddies, one wounded and being carried by his friend, who keeps talking to him in a frenzied effort to keep him alive. Eventually, the silence announces his death to the audience, but the friend just keeps talking, hoping against hope that his valiant efforts to get his friend to safety have worked. And finally, the closing scene of the film shows the main character, a young and good-looking man, stretch out to a butterfly that has landed on the barbed wire, a fleeting echo of the possibility of beauty amidst the depravity, only to be killed by a sniper.

In this chapter I will discuss some specific outcomes of injuries that occur during childhood and these images serve as general context for the discussion. Four messages are reflected in the above cameo of warfare. These underpin my beliefs and attitudes concerning many of the human problems and experiences that I am going to examine here. Firstly, people can do the most terrible things to each other out of desperation, ignorance and conditioning. Secondly, we can judge and believe in the evil of others more easily as long as we don't know their story. Thirdly, loving friendship and support does not guarantee healing and recovery. And fourthly, human experiences, no matter how painful or grotesque, can be visited with the possibility of beauty.

The walking wounded are those who still have significant elements of their human spirit intact, but who carry wounds with them as they hobble, sometimes with great difficulty and pain, to find a way to live an authentic life. They search, and sometimes get very lost, for a way to live with themselves, seeking what all people in touch with their humanity look for: love, peace, joy and a sense of meaning and purpose.

There are at least six major ways in which people who have been injured in childhood express these injuries in adulthood. These are: 1. violence; 2. co-dependency; 3. addiction; 4. emotional disorder; 5. Religiosity/ideology; and 6. the abuse of power. Each of these patterns for living in the world can interweave, to create a constellation of destructive feelings and behaviour that may be unique to each individual.

Violence

The cable of violence has many strands and, of all human experiences, it becomes one of the most contentious when we begin to try to explain its nature and its causes. In general, human violence can be divided into three major categories. Firstly, outbursts of rage, sometimes unprovoked; secondly, calculated and premeditated efforts to hurt and/or kill oneself or others for some purpose other than the violence itself; and thirdly, calculated and premeditated efforts to hurt and/or kill oneself or others for the sake of hurting or killing them.

The first category is less complex than the latter two. Outbursts of rage occur in people who have a low tolerance for frustration, a store of unresolved anger towards others and in many cases an experience of receiving violent punishment or ill-treatment in childhood. Most familial violence fits into this category (and in the modern world, most violence is familial). This category of violence has the most relevance to the theme of this book. Growing up within a dysfunctional family creates a great deal of anger in some children. The unfairness, disrespect and cruelty that are the hallmarks of many such families leave dark crevices of bitterness and rage in the heart of the growing child, often further exacerbated within the school, as people react to his anger; the young individual gradually becomes a walking 'time-bomb'.

Carrying out a seemingly normal life, this individual may convince those outside his intimate circle that they are reasonably intact. Those close to them know otherwise. They may swing from periods of intense anger, including verbal and sometimes physical assault, to feelings of deep remorse. Promising never to do it again and trying to make amends, they often are deeply upset by their truly behaviour. Then, as the pressure mounts again, something small and seemingly trivial triggers off his explosive anger and once again they leave in their wake an after wash of devastated feelings in partners and children. This type of violence is best described by Alice Miller as the 'compulsion to repeat'. The person is unconsciously repeating what happened to them at a time when they were helpless, and is also driven by the unresolved rage that had been buried as they endured the abuse of others as a child. (It is important to emphasis that not everyone who has endured violence in their formative years becomes violent. And it is not to excuse or justify their behaviour) This person is one of the walking wounded. He or she is often quite a sensitive individual and may have many good and worthwhile qualities. The torment they bring to their own life and the lives of others is an expression of his unhealed wounds. With proper care and attention to these, they can find healing and recovery.

The second type of violence is far more complex and difficult to deal with. It involves the person's belief system as well as his unresolved emotional issues. In this case, the violence is seen as purposeful. Violence against others is used as an instrument for getting what one wants. Killing a bank clerk during a robbery, stabbing someone during a mugging and blowing innocent people to bits with a bomb are all examples of utilitarian forms of violence. The latter example of terrorism is even more complex, in that it involves a perversion of values, rather than a simple denial of such values. In all cases, the core of this kind of violence is the belief that the victims are in some way less important than the goal which the perpetrator has set for himself. While there are deep and complex social and political forces involved in this form of violence, I am convinced that the basic root - the diminishment of the value of human beings - is often a result of childhood influences. Whenever we demean or abuse a child, we sow a seed and create a valence for them to be able, with greater ease, to act violently as adults. These people are far more likely to embrace cults, parties and political movements that validate or legitimize cruelty and persecution of others.

The third form of violence is violence for its own sake. This is not strictly accurate, for no one is violent purely for itself, but for the emotional rather than practical outcomes. I am reminded here of C.S. Lewis' lucid comment that:

... wickedness, when you examine it, turns out to be the pursuit of some good in the wrong way. You can be good for the mere sake of goodness: you cannot be bad for the mere sake of badness. You can do a kind action when you are not feeling kind and when it gives you no pleasure, simply because kindness is right, but no one ever did a cruel action simply because cruelty is wrong - only because cruelty was pleasant or useful to him. In other words, badness cannot succeed even in being bad in the same way in which goodness is good. Goodness is, so to speak, itself: badness is only spoiled- goodness. And there must be something good first before it can he spoiled.

There is a flaw in this argument in that if you do a cruel act because it is pleasurable to do so then we have to take a step back and ask why does the person find it pleasant to be cruel.

Many examples of violence, both physical and verbal, appear purposeless, in so far as no external practical ends seem to be served by it. We can, however, gain a clearer understanding of violence and the person who uses it when we look more closely at the emotional gains that are made. I should say here that such understanding provides us with the reasons why much violence occurs, but it does not excuse it. Most sexual violence, both inside and outside marriage, fits into this category. The perpetrator uses sex as a weapon and gratifies his need for dominance, power and revenge. These are the payoffs to the perpetrator, not the sexual act itself. Then there are people who express great violence against themselves, often cutting themselves because of inner turmoil. Their internal pain can find no expression, and there is a sense of satisfaction and release when they draw the razor over their bodies. Another form of seemingly purposeless violence is defensive violence. Many people are physically or verbally violent as a reaction to feeling threatened, even when, to an onlooker, this threat seems minimal. Most animals run away when threatened, until they find themselves cornered, when they attack. People, it seems, share this characteristic. Those who have experienced violence, when allied with a tendency to feel easily threatened, run a high risk of becoming violent adults.

The clearest and most extreme example of this type of violence is that of serial killing. Those who kill people regularly for no apparent motive are often operating violently from a sick and evil set of internal influences. Others appear to be driven by both their interior demons and the need to make some kind of quasi-religious or existential statement. In this context, one thinks of the hellish marriage of the paranoia of the Yorkshire ripper and the alienated and estranged Raskolnikov in Dostoyevsky's Crime and

Punishment. Whatever this dreadful mix, we can be sure of one thing: the presence of a tight line of hatred that underlies all of these acts. Whether this is self-hatred or hatred of another, we can also be sure that such depth of hatred cannot arrive in a heart that has been cultivated and encouraged to love. And, thus, we are back to the beginning, the foundation of life - the formative years of childhood.

Violence, then, in all its forms involves the abuse and demeaning of human beings. In all of this, there is no suggestion that an individual is not responsible for how he or she chooses to act out of his or her internal turmoil. Rather, these explanations help us to understand that the roots of violence always lie in the heart of the perpetrators. And, furthermore, the vulnerability of a human being to the scars of abuse and diminishment is vastly increased during the years of youth. Brian Keenan, in his book An Evil Cradling, provides an eloquent and perhaps fitting summary for this section by saying:

"Cruelty and fear are man-made, and men who perpetrate them are ruled by them. Such men are only half-made things. They live out their unresolved lives by attempting to destroy anything that challenges the void in themselves. A child holds a blanket over its face in fear. A fear-filled man transposes his inadequacy on to another. He blames them, hates them, and hopes to rid himself of his unloved self by hurting, or worse, destroying them".

As I write this I can hear the cynical voice of those who complain that here again we have the psychologist trotting out the tired old excuse for violent behaviours, it's the fault of a bad childhood. I can well understand this complaint because there is a great deal of violence in the world that does not have its roots in childhood trauma. In a recent book "The Path to Mass Evil" I show how a whole society can be encouraged and influenced to become violent collaborators and perpetrators, and this has very little to do with childhood influences. It has to do with ideological corruption. This does not invalidate the argument here that some human violence is perpetrated directly as a result of the emotional damage caused in childhood.

Co-dependency

Another pattern that grows out of the injuries of childhood is that of co-dependency. In some ways, co-dependency is a subtle form of violence against oneself. It involves several key concepts. These are: a low self-esteem; a high tolerance for suffering; a need to define one's worth in terms of other people's opinions; an overestimation of the suffering of others; an underestimation of others' ability to help themselves; and a sense of failure when one cannot make somebody else happy or 'fix' them. All of these add up to a severe form of dysfunction in terms of how to relate to oneself and others, particularly those close to us.

It could also be said that co-dependency is a feature of many personal relationships' and is often encouraged within our present views of relationships, particularly those of intimate partnerships. And, for all its apparent normality, co-dependency is a mind-numbing, emotionally crippling, life-threatening condition. Whilst men are more likely to express childhood injury through violence, women are more likely to suffer from co-dependency.

Low self-esteem is the beginning of co-dependency. This occurs in childhood when the child is treated badly; that is, when he or she is unsupported, unloved and given little of what he or she needs in terms of affection, admiration, praise and guidance. Some children will, as a result of these deficiencies, externalise their self-esteem into relationships. This means that they become completely dependent on the valuation of others in order to feel good about themselves.

We have seen that the periods of childhood and adolescence have, as their purpose, the formation of people whose sense of identity is intact and who have a high level of love and respect for themselves. Without these positive formative influences, a person can wander through life desperately searching for somebody to give them that sense of self-esteem. As a result, such a person becomes a hostage to anyone who responds with praise or affection. When a co-dependent person makes contact with another person, he or she is immediately watchful, checking to see what kind of impression is being made. On sensing any dislike/rejection on the part of the contacted person, he or she will go to great lengths to change that person's impression to a positive one. Once that has been achieved, the co-dependent moves on to the next contact, always on the look-out for that special person who holds the cure for his or her internal angst. A client of mine recently told me a story that nicely illustrates this. The story goes thus: a co-dependent goes into a bar where there are ten others gathered. Nine of the ten feel positively toward him and one doesn't. An hour later after valiant efforts to get the negative person to like him there is one person who is positive toward him and nine who have lost their earlier good disposition. He related it to me because he felt it resonated so much with his own life.

Co-dependent people learn early to accept that which is unacceptable. They learn not to expect a lot from others, and are surprised when someone has a positive attitude to them. More extreme forms of co-dependency lead to a rejection of love, because the person is unable to cope with or trust it. This can lead to a flaw that is often fatal to relationships, namely, a need continually to test the sincerity of a lover's commitment until he or she walks away, only reinforcing the co-dependent's view that the love and acceptance weren't real in the first place.

Paradoxically, then, co-dependents can be impossible to please, because they cannot trust that they are loved or valued. It is sometimes easier for them to live with those who show them little love or respect, because that is what they are familiar with; this also leaves them continually challenged to make the one who treats them badly change in attitude. In other cases, it is not unusual for a co-dependent person to marry the first person who shows any real interest in him or her, on that basis alone. In either situation, the co-dependent is left struggling for years in a relationship that from the outset did not have what he or she needed. A pithy definition I came across recently describes co-dependency as a condition that involves getting you needs met by not getting your needs met.

Ahigh tolerance for suffering and the capacity for endurance often, then, lead to a life of unhappiness and stress. This makes relationships with others fragile and frightening. Fear plays a significant part in co-dependent relationships. The stakes are very high - the needs for love and acceptance are intense, but these are bounded by an equally intense fear of rejection. This leads to the second strand of co-dependency: a need to define one's worth in terms of the opinions of others.

Co-dependent people do not have a secure sense of their own identity. They look outside themselves for a basis on which to gauge their worth. It is extremely difficult for them to risk rejection or criticism. This leads to perfectionistic behaviour and a high level of self-criticism. As a consequence, co-dependents set very high standards for themselves, are usually very responsible and hard-working, and will do any thing rather than risk failure in their own eyes or those of their colleagues and friends.

A second element in this area is the difficulty which co-dependents experience in making any decision that might discomfort someone else. Lack of assertiveness is, therefore, an intrinsic part of co-dependency. The risk involved in saying 'no' to a request is, for a co-dependent, great indeed. This combination means that co-dependents take on too much responsibility, are perfectionistic in trying to carry out their commitments and rarely, if ever, count the cost to their own health and happiness. This pattern means that they are likely to be excellent workers, until they finally explode or become ill from the perceived pressure under which they put themselves. Thus, in addition to the problems that are encountered in their personal relationships, a new burden of pressure arises in the way that they cope with their working lives. And, as if all this isn't enough to undo them, they have a predilection to become involved in areas of work that are by their nature very draining of their emotional resources. This comes about as a result of a third strand of co-dependency: an attraction to those who suffer.

Co-dependent people overestimate the suffering of others and underestimate people's ability to do anything about it. It is this aspect that leads so many co-dependents into the caring professions. When this happens, the co-dependent is setting themselves up for a stressful and over-demanding working life. This is ironic, in that co-dependents are the very people who have least resources really to offer help to others without exhausting their own meagre emotional and spiritual resources. Overestimating the struggles of others occurs by projecting one's own unhappiness onto them (i.e. seeing one's own unhappiness in others). Having experienced so much turmoil and pain in their early life, co-dependent people are keenly aware of what suffering feels like. It is, therefore, only a short step for them to believe that, when they see someone else in pain, it is like the pain that they have felt, but which lies underground and unresolved in the psyche.

By 'helping' others, co-dependents are indirectly trying to help themselves. This 'transference' usually occurs unconsciously, in that co-dependents are unaware that it is their own unresolved pain that they see reflected in the suffering of others. By becoming a healer of that pain, they are indirectly trying to heal their own pain. The greater the intensity of suffering that they have repressed, the more acute is the reaction to observing pain in others.

Allied to this is the belief again often unconscious - that a suffering person is helpless to do anything about it. This belief is grounded in the co-dependent's own experiences of helplessness when, in childhood, he or she was powerless to change the suffering inflicted on him or her in the family. Many grew up in families where their daily experience included not only a personally painful environment, but also an everyday routine of watching one or both parents, and perhaps their siblings, suffer in what appeared to them un resolvable and unending turmoil. Small wonder, then, that when presented with the reality of suffering in others they impose the message of childhood: that these people are as helpless as those who peopled their earliest memories.

And finally, this complex web of emotional traps is completed with an element of co-dependency that leads many who suffer in this way to a lifetime of futility. This is their overweening sense of responsibility for the happiness of others. Co-dependent people are often afflicted with enormous guilt in relation to how others feel. This guilt is grounded in an overdeveloped sense of responsibility for others. In their family of origin, many co-dependents were emotionally blackmailed and made to feel that the struggle and toil of their parents was somehow related to the child's existence. This message may have been made directly by parents, or indirectly by being exposed to the suffering of the parents.

Children, we now realise, are prone to seeing everything in terms of themselves. This is a healthy part of development when they are growing up in a safe, secure, and loving environment. Many of those who find themselves in traumatic or unhappy families are, however, immediately disposed to blame themselves, and to take responsibility for trying to fix those who are troubled in the family. In adulthood, these people tend to blame themselves for the feelings of others, and believe that they have somehow failed when their efforts to make that person happy haven't succeeded. Conversely, when such efforts do prove of value to others, co-dependents tend to take credit for the change, and continue in the trap of externalising their self-worth by making it conditional on the degree to which they make others feel good. They are also far more likely to be attracted to relationship swith people who have the opposite problem, an insatiable need to use others for their own ends. This is the phenomenon of Narcissism.

Narcissism

The term 'Narcissist' comes from ancient mythology. The function of myth making in ancient cultures was to help people make sense of life. These stories are timeless because they carry moral insights into the various struggles and flaws that inhere human nature. The myth of Narcissus is one case in point and is particularly relevant to the present discussion of self-worth. In the classical myth Narcissus was a hunter who was renowned for both his beauty as well as his scorn for those who loved him. Nemesis, the goddess of divine retribution, seeing this flaw, led Narcissus to a clear pool where he could see his reflection plainly. He so fell in love with himself that he lost all other interest and eventually wasted away and died.

The important element in this myth for the current discussion lies in the fate of Narcissus. He wasted away. People who are filled with self-aggrandisement and snobbery also waste away. Their lives are ultimately empty. Part of this emptiness occurs because they are unable to partake in some of the most nourishing and enriching experiences open to a human being; the main one being that of intimacy. Narcissists are incapable of intimacy.To experience the enrichment of the soul by opening and meeting the soul of another is impossible for a narcissistic person. This is because all their interactions with other are focussed on using the other person for their own ends. These ends include attention seeking, using others resources to enhance their own position in ways that support their vanity, this can include using others for status, for financial gain, for security.

They also fail to grow spiritually. By this I mean being able to experience the self-transcendent conditions of deep love, appreciation of beauty, being transported by the sense of connection to a higher being, or higher power through music, prayer or engagement with nature.

Narcissistic people are also likely to be destructive of others. They are prone to what is called narcissistic rage, which is provoked by anything that is perceived as a threat to their self-importance. Narcissists use others while at the same time being incapable of empathy. Empathy is that human capacity for understanding at a cognitive and emotional level the experience of others, to see and feel the world from another's viewpoint. Empathy is an essential aspect of any close human bond. Their relationships are thus superficial and manipulative and those who engage with them gradually feel more and more helpless as they try valiantly to gain approval and love from someone who has none to give.

All of these strands lead to an emotionally devastating way of living. In all major areas of life, including relationship to self, others and to work, co-dependents are slowly spinning into a vortex of emotional, spiritual and intellectual exhaustion. Small wonder, then, that many find themselves gradually entrapped by either addiction or emotional disorder. It is to these issues we now turn.

Addiction

Perhaps the most visible examples of the walking wounded are those who have fallen prey to some form of addiction. In this section I will discuss several specific addictions, namely: drug addiction (including alcoholism); compulsive gambling; addiction to sex; and addiction to work. My discussion will, of necessity, be brief. (A more detailed discussion of addiction can be found in another book of mine. Understanding Addiction. A Common sense Approach.) My main objective here is to outline the destructive nature of these addictions. Other similar phenomena include addiction to food, excitement and certain forms of relationship. Each of these addictions has its own specific features, but they all share certain common themes.

Addiction, in most cases, is the abuse of any substance or activity that leads to self-destruction. The core element of addiction, in my opinion, is the individual's use of such substances or activities to achieve one or more of the following purposes: filling a void or sense of emptiness; quelling distressing feelings; and/or producing pleasant and euphoric sensations.

Once addiction takes hold of an individual, his or her day-to-day life reflects certain patterns of behaviour that further exacerbate these problems. In general, there is moral, social, physical and emotional deterioration. Telling lies, for example, becomes an intrinsic part of the addict's weaponry of denial. Manipulation of others leads to secrecy, dishonesty, crooked thinking and the use and abuse of others. Morally, the person begins to act in ways often unthinkable during his or her pre-addiction life; examples of this abound, and include: stealing; borrowing with no intention of paying back; setting up others to enable and help the addiction, with no concern for their welfare; and abusive blaming of others in order to deflect interest in his or her increasingly chaotic lifestyle. Destructive behaviour, ranging from outbursts of rage (described above), to suicidal tendencies, ruthless coldness and disregard for relationships all become staging posts on the downward slope to eventual death, if recovery is not instituted.

The most commonly recognised addiction is that of drug addiction. There are three basic forms of this disorder: addiction to alcohol; addiction to prescribed drugs; and addiction to illegal street drugs. The central feature of each of these is a chemical dependency, allied to a psychological need for the effects of the drug on the mind and emotions. Many influences are at work in determining the type of drug that becomes the user's drug of choice. One issue that needs clarification here is that whilst people who are damaged in childhood can react to this damage by turning to drugs to anaesthetize their internal turmoil, this does not mean that all people who misuse drugs have had an unhappy or traumatic family of origin. Some otherwise healthy individuals, for example, will have experimented with drugs as part of adolescent rebellion and become addicted. Others, in adult life, may turn to drugs to help cope with some of the normal stresses and strains of life. I believe, however, based on my experience of working with recovering addicts, that the majority of drug addicts are people who are carrying wounds from their formative years.

Alcoholism is the most prevalent drug addiction in western society. And the evidence to date suggests that it is at least as devastating a condition as more sensational forms of drug abuse. Most 'alcoholics' (or problem drinkers) begin drinking in their late teens, and it takes an average of ten years for the addiction to take complete hold of the individual. There is usually a progression from social drinking into heavy problem drinking and then on to full-blown addiction. The turning point in each of these stages is usually unclear, but we do know that one of the signposts of addiction is the deepening chemical dependence, which announces its presence in the form of withdrawal symptoms when the drug is absent. These withdrawal symptoms can be so severe that a person may die if left without medical intervention, which usually means muscle relaxant and sedating medication. The dreadful consequences of withdrawal tell us of the profound physical as well as psychological nature of alcohol addiction.

Addiction to prescribed drugs also presents a severe form of disorder. Perhaps the most common form of this addiction is the dependence -both emotional and physical - that occurs in the long-term use of anti-anxiety medication. Once hailed as miracle drugs, the benzodiazepines are now recognised as extremely dangerous. By nature, these drugs - commonly called tranquillizers and/or sleeping pills - are tolerance forming. This means that a person who takes them regularly needs higher and higher doses in order to maintain their sedating effects. Furthermore, while doing nothing to solve the underlying anxiety for which they are used, they produce greater levels of anxiety when a person tries to reduce or stop their intake. In general, then, they create more problems for the user, and do little or nothing to solve the problems for which they are prescribed. As addiction develops, the person becomes increasingly less able to cope even with mundane tasks. A host of side-effects become more and more apparent, including slurred speech, drowsiness, mental deterioration, emotional blunting, muscular pains and spasms, sexual dysfunction and many others.

Addiction to illegal street drugs is the third major form of drug abuse. I am including here the abuse of solvents, even though they are not illegal. Generally, these drugs can be categorised in terms of the type and intensity of their effects. Certain well-known compounds are primarily hallucinogenic in nature. This means that they produce altered states of consciousness, with many visual and auditory images and sensations. Mescaline, LSD, magic mushrooms and ecstasy are the more familiar drugs in this category.

Addiction to these is primarily psychological. An individual who uses these drugs finds everyday reality more and more difficult to live in, and increasingly turns to the new realities produced by the drugs in order to cope. These drugs have enormous potential to damage thinking processes, and can lead to psychoses. Other well-known drugs are those that are termed opiates and their derivatives. These include heroin, morphine and methadone (which is used to wean heroin addicts from their primary drug). These drugs mimic the production of natural pain killers called endorphins, and are extremely addictive. There is powerful physical, as well as psychological, dependency associated with this category of drug. Finally, cannabis is the most popular of the street drugs; many argue that it should be decriminalized, as it is less addictive and less harmful than nicotine. Much contention exists on both sides of this argument.

My own view is that regardless of what mood-altering substances are legal, there will be a significant number of people who will abuse them (tranquillizer addiction is a good case in point). Cocaine and its cheaper, chemically synthesized, counterpart called crack are other well-known illegal drugs. Until recently, the former was the drug of choice of the more economically well off. Part of the mythology of its use is that it isn't physically addictive. Cocaine is in fact an extremely dangerous drug and crack is even more deadly. The capacity of these drugs to take psychological hold on a person is now recognised, as well as their toxic and often fatal effects on the body.

Untreated drug addiction, including alcoholism, usually leads to death. The walking wounded frequently exacerbate many of the injuries that lie within themselves by turning to drugs and, as a result, many never recover. Perhaps the most poignant, and dramatic, account of the slavery and futility of this endeavour is recounted by Danny Sugerman in his book *Wonderland Avenue: Tales of Glamour and Excess*. His involvement with the music scene, and the group The Doors, brought him at a very young age into the maelstrom of the drug culture of the 1960s. Sugerman's account is a useful and poetic way to conclude this section. Towards the end of his story of drug addiction (and a lot else), and having begun to count the cost to himself and the loss of so many of his friends who died, he says:

Jesus. The first thing I wanted to do was find the jerk who invented the saying 'if it feels good, do it', and then go after the bozo who started the rumour that drugs enhance creativity, tie them both to the nearest tree and blow their fucking brains out. Yeah, okay, fine, then what? What about all your buddies? What about Arthur Rimbaud? What about Baudelaire? And Artaud? What about Coleridge and Cocteau? And Byron? What about James Dean. And Jimi Hendrix? What about all of them? What about all the others you love so much? ... They died of addiction and disease and madness and they died long before their prime... I think the best feeling they knew was the feeling of relief. That's what these once glorious men were reduced to. Pain didn't inspire them anymore. It overwhelmed them, engulfed them and ate them up alive. They were not strong enough or smart enough to fight it, to deal with it, or beat it. It obsessed them shame fully, pitifully and completely. Would any of them say, 'Look at me, hold me up as an example to the young and impressionable of the world because I led a good and courageous life. I drank and drugged myself to death and I'm glad I did it and I'm glad my life is over.' Would any single one of these guys say, 'I like death better than living?' You're godammed right they wouldn't. And were they to speak to us today, if they were really so goddamn brave and true and honest, they'd admit it. They'd tell us what it was really like. They died crying in their minds like little babies, lonely and afraid, yearning for the face of a friend. They died depressed and sick, wanting another look at the sun or the seashore; they wanted again to hear the voice of a mother, a father, a lover or a child. They died moaning and sighing for life. Because in the end they knew what was really important. They died with one thought only in their minds, and that thought was: I want to live, I want to live, I want to live... And it's harder and braver to live than it is to die. Dying is easy. It's living that takes real courage ... What the fuck was I looking for, anyway? What was so goddamn all-important? Freedom? What's so liberating about becoming a slave? And what good is freedom if you use it to kill yourself? I'm sorry, but there's nothing glamorous about being an addict. There's nothing noble about a rotting liver; nothing heroic about a rotting corpse. A heart attack at twenty-seven years old? Like Morrison? Or dead at twenty-one? Me, I want to live. You know what I think Morrison would have said? 'Experience, feel the pain. Without pain there is no change. Without change there is no growth, and if you don't grow you die. Don't make the same mistakes I made. Make different ones. Don't be stupid. Grow. Live.'

Gambling is a less well-known addiction. For many people, the notion that someone can become addicted to gambling seems unlikely. It seems rather strange that a person can feel tremendous craving and a powerful compulsion to bet on a horse or spend hours in front of a poker machine. To a clear-thinking person, such behaviour seems rather easy to avoid if one wishes to. Gambling addiction is, however, a much more complex business than simply wanting badly to take betting risks. It is also hugely destructive. The obvious damage that is incurred financially is often reflective of equally destructive emotional, spiritual and intellectual destruction.

The intricate nature of gambling addiction is not well understood, because it has only been recognised as a serious disorder in recent years. Several elements are emerging, how ever, which tend to be an underlying part of the disorder. Gambling addicts for the most part tend to deal with emotional distress by using defensive mechanisms of distraction and rationalisation. In other words, like other types of addicts, they have a lot of problems coping with their feelings. What tends to set them apart is their use of thinking as a means of avoidance. Once this pattern is established, they are prime candidates for gambling problems. Having tasted the experience of gambling, they have been presented with a situation that can utilise all their mental energy. The risks inherent in betting occupy the mind and eventually take it over completely. Allied to this is the adrenaline surge inherent in the excitement of the risk of winning or losing.

Gradually, a cycle of obsessional thinking about gambling takes a firmer and firmer hold on the person's mind. Emotionally exhausted from the outcome of this addiction, he or she has less and less resources to attend to his or her relationships, family and work. As financial problems mount, the individual becomes more secretive and deceitful, mort gaging an increasing amount of resources in the growing difficulties of losing greater sums of money, all the while hoping for the big win that will relieve this burden. Should this win occur, he or she is likely to lose it all again - and so the cycle continues. Most untreated gambling addicts eventually lose everything they own - and often a lot of what they don't own- leading to life-long debt and financial impoverishment. Emotional withdrawal follows, with deeper anxiety sometimes leading to suicide, or turning to some other addictive substance such as alcohol. Within a period of years, the person becomes an emotional and spiritual wreck.

Even more recent is the discovery that people can become addicted to sexual conquest. It may be that sexual addiction is a relatively new phenomenon, or that it has always existed and is only now coming to light. My own view is that addictions in general are culture bound, which means that people tend to become addicted to substances and activities that have some cultural license. Thus, for example, the Japanese are more likely to become addicted to amphetamines, the Chinese to opiates and the Irish to alcohol. The sexual revolution of the 1960s and 70s has now established itself as a more liberal and permissive view of sexual behaviour. Casual sex is a social reality in most western societies. Certain people who are inclined toward addiction, for the reasons described above, are now more likely to find a way of expressing this addictive tendency in sexual relationships.

Like most addictions, sexual addiction has certain defining characteristics. Sex addicts are compulsively engaged in the use of sexual conquest for emotional distraction and relief. Their sexual contacts have little, if anything, to do with intimacy or relationship. Nor have they anything to do with the relatively normal sexual needs that some people express by having a number of sexual encounters, particularly during their young adulthood. Rather, sex addiction is a compulsively driven need to make sexual conquests very regularly. The main feature of these engagements is that they are used to fulfil the addict's sense of inner emptiness, or to alleviate feelings of anxiety or distress. Many sex addicts have been sexually molested as children. Those who become addictive in their sexual behaviour tend to choose sexual partners who they 'know' will use and abandon them. For many such people, there is an enormous confusion between sex and love, with the former often considered to be the only way to receive the latter. In certain cases, there is also the issue of revenge. Some prostitutes, for example, have a hatred of men and operate their sexuality out of this underlying feeling. The role of hatred and revenge is, however, particularly important in understanding male sex addiction. The rather crude adage: find them, feel them, use them and forget them is for male sex addicts the underlying attitude to women. In those cases where anger and revenge are a feature of the addiction, much of the childhood influences have occurred as a result of witnessing an abusive relationship between the parents or receiving abusive treatment from the parent of the opposite sex.

Perhaps the most socially condoned and approved addiction is that which relates to work. Like co-dependency, it is a very common disorder which, on the outside, appears normal; its effects, however, are very destructive to any form of healthy, balanced life. Workaholics are those people whose existence becomes completely dominated by work. Many of the elements of other addictions described above also play a part in work addiction and do not need to be repeated here. One aspect that appears to be specific to this form of addiction, though, is the need to secure the future through accumulation of wealth or assets. Work addicts are, in general, fearful of financial ruin, and many, through their great need to accumulate, take major financial risks and end up in financial trouble.

Insecurity is then a strong element in work addiction. Those close to the addict experience the loss of present-day security in the relationship, as the addict tries to make the future secure for his family. Many workaholics have come from backgrounds where there was financial worry, sometimes as a result of parental addiction, such as alcoholism. In their effort 'never to experience this again', they end up ruining their health and happiness through overwork.

Another strong element in workaholism is that of pride. Having experienced conditional love as a child, many work addicts believe that their worth is based on their career success and on the amount of money they make. Even as the wealth accumulates, the work addict cannot enjoy its benefits. Deeply unhappy within, money cannot buy peace of mind, love or fulfilment. Each job well done and each substantial financial gain only give a fleeting sense of satisfaction which must be repeated again and again. A stranger to his partner and children, the work addict strives ever harder to find that elusive feeling of being a worthwhile human being.

As the years roll on, the person gets more and more frustrated. Perhaps they experience a traumatic mid-life crisis, underpinned by the recognition of reduced energy and by being overtaken by those younger. In this case, the individual is prey to other forms of addiction, to sexual acting out or to major depression. The degree to which these storms are weathered are significant indications as to whether some form of physical or mental crisis will eventually overtake the person, leading to early death, suicide or emotional breakdown.

Emotional Problems

Thus far we have examined certain behaviours that become part of a person's destructive lifestyle. Each of these are identifiable as consistent patterns of behaving which grow out of internal distress. Emotional disorders are more closely related to the internal state of the individual. Three major emotional disorders are: depression;

anxiety; and obsessive-compulsive reactions. Depression and anxiety are clinical words used to describe chronic feelings of sadness and fearfulness experienced by a person. Obsessive-compulsive reactions is a disorder that combines an emotional state of fearfulness with some kind of compulsive thinking, or way of acting. Each of these disorders is a symptom of underlying conflict, which is often a result of damaging experiences that occurred in early life during the person's formation.

Depression is considered the common cold of the mental disorders. Millions of people worldwide are treated each year for its appearance in their lives. Many books are written to help people cope with it and millions of pounds are spent on a variety of drugs for use in its treatment. In this section, I will briefly examine the phenomenon. My primary aim is to show how depression can be an outcome of early experience, and thus can be reversed and avoided through the process of recovery discussed in the next part of this book.

Sadness is a normal human emotion; it provides us with a means of healing our hurts and dealing with our losses. Its presence in our lives becomes a disorder when it appears and continues for no apparent reason, or when it remains an intrinsic part of our experience long after the event which gave rise to it. When this happens, it is usually called depression. The experience of depression has several elements. It is an emotional state which combines feelings of sadness, loneliness, emotional numbness, helplessness and hopelessness. The depressed person finds living difficult; sexual and eating disorders often follow. Everything in life seems negative, and carrying on is a great effort. There is little joy in anything, including relating to others - particularly those close to the depressed person. Warmth and intimacy are only fleeting experiences, if they occur at all. Generally, the person feels as if he or she has fallen into an emotional pit and is swimming through treacle each grey and lonely day.

There are many causes of depression, and many theories that try to explain its origin and treatment. Here I am confining the discussion to those aspects of depression that appear to have their roots in childhood. Three underlying elements in most depression are particularly relevant in this regard: a sense of loss; an unexpressed anger; and a feeling of helplessness. As we have seen, these are often very real experiences in the life of a child growing up in a dysfunctional family.

The most common and debilitating sense of loss is the loss of self-worth and self-esteem. The failure to develop a healthy and positive self-image is almost always a result of childhood influences. Conditional love, lack of affection, high levels of criticism and punishment lead the growing person into a fundamental belief in his own unworthiness. This core attitude to oneself is very difficult to shake off as an adult. As a consequence, many people who experience themselves in this negative way have already lost a hugely important part of their well-being. When other losses occur on the journey of life, the ghosts of these early losses are awoken and can cause great emotional distress and pain. The emotional trauma of many events lies not in the events themselves, but in their capacity to stir old wounds from the slumber of the unconscious and to attach themselves to present-day experience. Thus, those who were emotionally abandoned in early life will again and again feel intense feelings of loss when they lose relationships or other important aspects of their lives as adults. This often results in depression.

Another aspect of depression is unresolved anger. Many people who experience depression have great difficulty expressing anger. Like sadness, anger is a normal human emotion. In its healthy expression, it helps us to protect our selves and to fight for what we need. Many children who grow up in dysfunctional homes have the fight knocked out of them. Not only have they lost a great deal in terms of self-worth, they have also been trained not to express negative feelings and to avoid conflict at all costs. Some of these children are sensitive in temperament and therefore more prone to internalize their anger. This means that they are more inclined to blame themselves, and become critical and punitive towards themselves rather than risk the trauma of fighting back. In adulthood, when new losses occur, these people end up blaming themselves and becoming harsh in their attitude to themselves. This combines with an already low self-image to bring the person down even further. These two elements, of low self-esteem and an inability to fight for one's needs and protection, lead to a third strand of depression - that of a helpless-hopeless outlook on life.

A person's ability to cope with everyday life can be gradually eroded to the point where he or she feels unable to go on. When this happens, the prospect of suicide becomes frightfully close as a means of leaving this place of pain and sadness. Underlying this attraction to death is a belief that nothing one does makes any difference, and that things will not get any better. What many in this emotional state do not realise is that it is not life that is hopeless, but that one's confidence and optimism have become so withered that opportunities for change are avoided or let go, leading to further feelings of failure and hopelessness. These feelings can be extremely intense, to the point where a person stops being able to function at all. The world comes to be seen through a tunnel of despair. Changes of thinking occur, and all experience of life is seen as a burden to be borne. Relationships die, as the individual can no longer give or receive the emotional care and attention needed to sustain them. This exacerbates the already pessimistic outlook on life, by leaving the individual lonely and feeling unloved. All of these changes are occurring internally, and recovery involves serious changes in how the person thinks and acts in the world. It is only then that the awful feelings will gradually dissipate, to be replaced by new, more positive, and life-enhancing ones. (This issue is addressed in the next chapter.)

A second, very common, emotional disorder is that of anxiety. Rather than depend on this rather clinical term, I prefer to use the word fearfulness. In general, this state is marked by feelings of tension and fear that appear to have no specific origin or object. Some people who suffer in this way are likely to feel frightened most of the time, but cannot find a reason why. Each day is marked by physical feelings that include palpitations, sweating, shivering and a host of other fear-induced bodily experiences. Psychologically, the individual is visited by dread and apprehension. It's as if at any moment catastrophe is going to occur, and yet there is no obvious reason to expect such disastrous outcomes in each ordinary day.

Other people develop phobias. These are unreasonable fears that lead to panic in situations that are to most people unthreatening. Examples of this phenomenon abound, and have clinical names like agoraphobia (fear of crowded places, e.g. supermarkets and busy streets); claustrophobia (fear of small enclosed spaces - lifts, small rooms, etc.); acrophobia (fear of heights, multi-storey buildings, cliffs, bridges, etc.); and a myriad of others. There are very specific treatments available for this kind of phobic fearfulness. I am inclined toward the view, however, that people who become phobic are fearful in general. The phobia is an expression of this fearfulness. This happens when the fear becomes attached to a specific object, usually after some traumatic incident involving that object. An example is where someone runs out of money at a supermarket check-out, leading to a fear of supermarkets that then generalises to other busy places.

Fearfulness is often a legacy of having grown up in a destructive family environment. In this regard, there are two key elements in such fearfulness: vigilance and powerlessness. Vigilance refers to the expectation of danger. Children who are wounded in their family of origin have learned early on that one way of coping within the family is to become watchful for signs that tell that danger is on the way. This is most clearly seen in alcoholic homes, where the sound of the key in the door is sufficient for children to brace themselves for the verbal or physical abuse that often follows. The outcome of living one's formative years in such an emotionally and sometimes physically dangerous environment is that one's psychological and physical make-up is often permanently affected. One of these effects is vigilance for danger. This can have devastating effects on one's functioning.

Our bodies are designed to react in special ways when we meet with danger. The fight or flight response is a built-in safety measure which helps us either to overcome or avoid danger. These safety mechanisms require a great deal of emotional energy, and are only rarely called upon in our lives, such as when we have to jump out of the way of a careering car, or when we grab a child before he falls off a wall, or when we run to be on time for a very important meeting. Fearful people live consistently in a state of preparedness for danger. This means that their bodies are tense and keyed up, often described as being 'highly strung', or 'wound up'.

The second element in fearfulness is that of powerlessness. Not only does the person continually brace themselves for possible danger, but also believes that they are powerless over it when it arrives. This sense of powerlessness is often based in the reality that as a child they could do nothing to prevent being hurt by his/her parents. Like many of those who suffer from depression, there is a loss of self-worth and self-confidence at the base of much fearfulness. Fearful people tend to see others as better or stronger than themselves, and at the same time see themselves as weaker and less able.

When, for example, a fearful person goes into a bank to negotiate a loan, they are already preparing for the danger of rejection and at the same time underestimating their ability to convince the bank representative of their value as a customer. Expecting rejection, he or she 'knows' that they will feel fearful in the encounter, so they brace themselves for dealing with being afraid. In some instances, the encounter will be avoided rather than confronted which will result in lower self-confidence and a failure to meet a financial need that could have led to a positive advance in their life. In the case where the decision to meet the bank personnel is progressed, they will not present as confident a case as they could, which may result in his not getting the loan. This further confirms a low view of himself and greater feelings of powerlessness.

Anxiety, or fearfulness, as discussed here can become a crippling condition. As an emotional disorder it is, in general, a symptom of deeper problems related to self-esteem, heightened sensitivity to danger and feelings of powerlessness. Recovery from this disorder needs to address these underlying problems.

A third major emotional disorder is that of obsessivecompulsive reactions. These refer to certain habits of either thinking or behaving that cause great distress for the suffering individual and often for those around him or her. The better-known examples of these are checking and cleanliness compulsions. Checking compulsions occur when a person is continually attacked by thoughts that he or she has not completed some activity such as locking doors, turning off cookers, lights and other electrical appliances. Once this thought springs to mind, the person feels anxious and begins to worry that the house will be burgled or burned down. After much self-torment, the person may return home, only to find everything as it should be. Within a short time of leaving, the doubts begin to creep in, leaving the person anxious and worried again.

Cleanliness compulsions are similar in nature, and occur when a person becomes intensely afraid of germs or contamination. Ritual handwashing, sometimes hundreds of times in a day, is an extreme example of this kind of compulsion. Cleaning door handles, clothes and appliances in order to get rid of germs are other well-known expressions of this disorder. Obsessional disorders are similar to compulsions, except that they are internal, mental events rather than outward expressions. Obsessions can be defined as a consistent focusing of a person's mental energy on some anxiety-producing facet of life. A good example is that of health obsession. In this instance, a person is obsessively concerned with his or her health. More specifically, there is an intense worry over some particular aspect, such as whether or not the person has cancer. Every ache and pain, whether real or imagined, is taken as evidence for the invasion of a tumour. When exhaustive tests prove negative, the individual begins to worry that perhaps he or she suffers from some new, unheard of disease.

Other examples of obsessions are those that afflict people who have strong religious beliefs. I have met individuals, particularly those who were exposed to very legalistic religious teaching, who worry greatly over whether or not they have made a proper confession of their sins. Before receiving communion, they rack their memories to check if any sins were not confessed and therefore are not forgiven. To receive communion while in a state of sin is, of course, in their belief a grave matter. People suffering with these obsessions are in torment, which they usually discuss with a priest, who eventually resorts to what is called a general absolution. This alleviates the problem for a short time, because it means that all sins committed - whether confessed or not - are absolved. This short-term solution gradually loses its impact as time moves on. The obsessional person accumulates more possible sins, and the cycle of moral anxiety continues, leading to greater torment.

Another form of this disorder is that of intrusive thoughts, usually of a horrible nature. Thoughts of killing one's children, stabbing one's spouse, or for the devout clergyman, masturbating into the chalice. These are that kind of uninvited and unwelcome thoughts that frighten the life out of the unfortunate sufferer who of course cannot tell anybody because they that believe that there is some intentional element in the thought. This can become an absolute nightmare if they attend a counsellor who looks for some hidden meaning in the thought and thereby give them some credence.

These disorders create havoc in a person's life, and also make life very difficult for those who are close to them. Two important elements underpin these problems: perfectionism and control. Some damaged children grow up into perfectionist adults. Usually as a result of experiencing conditional love on the one hand and fear of criticism and or rejection on the other, these people believe that they must be perfect in all things. As a result, they cannot compromise their standards and fail to learn one of the key strategies of health and maturity, namely adapting to the environment. Unable to compromise, they begin to drive themselves and those around them crazy with their detailed, exhaustive behaviour. Not only do they demand perfection from themselves, but they can also experience high levels of anger and frustration when others don't comply with their sense of order.

A second element is that of control. The perfectionist has a strong need to control his or her external environment, particularly the emotional states of those around him or her. Having never learned to deal adequately with the ebb and flow of his or her own emotional life, this person keeps his or her feelings under tight control. Rigid in personality, at an unconscious level he or she is terrified that all these feelings will spill uncontrollably into consciousness and wreak havoc. Anything in the environment that increases the likelihood that this may happen is subject to strict control.

Another form of this kind of control is found in the individual's compulsion to keep the environment in a very predictable order. Compulsive tidying, experiencing anxiety if something is out of order (a crooked picture for example), writing notes compulsively to help remember events, and sometimes notes about notes, all suggest a desperate need to keep order on the outside. In times of stress, these behaviours become more pronounced, sometimes to the point that the individual can no longer function. These people are also very prone to the problem of religiosity, a topic to which we now tum.

Religiosity

Almost a century ago, Freud wrote a book called The Future of an Illusion, suggesting that religion is a collective neurosis. A neurosis is a set of psychological defense mechanisms that a person develops in order to avoid anxiety. In Freud's view, the collective neurosis of most religion is the shared belief system that is used by particular societies in order to provide a means by which people can avoid the fear of death, the anxiety of aloneness and the pain of guilt. Much of the historical and anthropological foundation on which he built his ideas has since been discredited, but the central notion of religion as a set of mental defences has continued to gain acceptance in the field of psychology. My own view is that religion and spirituality are important aspects of human development. Like most aspects of our human nature, however, they can become destructive and dysfunctional.

Religiosity can be a refuge into which some people retreat in order to cope with the fragility of their lives. The outward expressions of religiosity are: intolerance for others of different beliefs; rigidity in personality - which means that the person has a overly strong need for rules and regulations; sexual dysfunction and lack of sensuality; a severe split between emotional and intellectual aspects of religious experience; a profound belief in the presence of evil in anything that does not agree with one's own religious viewpoint; a tendency to view most aspects of life as a struggle between good and evil; a critical, judgmental and sometimes patronising attitude towards others; an inability to cope with facts or experiences that do not fit with one's religious outlook; and a deep struggle with guilt. These and many other symptoms combine to create a very destructive way of life for some people.

Religiosity is a psychological rather than a spiritual phenomenon, and is underpinned by several personality characteristics that evolve from a damaged childhood. The more important of these are the need for certainty, repressed hostility and inability to trust. These characteristics attach themselves to religious (and sometimes political) concepts, and gradually provide a person with a survival strategy for making sense of life. This strategy creates more problems than it solves, leading to much distress for the individual and particularly for those close to him or her.

The need for certainty is an important element in religiosity. Thus, such people reach a position where they believe that they know the 'truth'. Anything that appears beyond their ability to understand is taken on faith. At a certain point, these individuals close their minds and hearts to new ways of understanding the world, and settle for a rigidly held set of religious mores and dogmas. Certainty is, of course, a very questionable virtue when it comes to the larger questions of life, such as the meaning of suffering, life after death, good and evil. Emotionally mature and healthy people continue to strive to understand these phenomena rather than settle for what is sometimes a very immature and childish set of beliefs. The growth of wisdom, in my opinion, is in proportion to the individual's willingness to question all things and to maintain some degree of openness to change. Those afflicted with religiosity miss the opportunity to become wise.

Hostility is also a part of religiosity. This element makes sense of the historical reality that great evil is carried out in the name of religion. In the present time, we can see all over the world tremendous brutality carried out under the banner of religious truth. In Ireland, the divisions between Roman Catholics and Protestants in the six counties of Ulster is a useful case in point. Hostility can easily be rationalised when a person believes that it is the will of the Divine to see people of another religion as lesser in God's eyes. Heretics bound for eternal punishment don't deserve equality of love, compassion and respect.

Lack of trust is also - and ironically - an element of most religiosity. The irony lies in the notion that trusting in God is usually one of the key stated virtues of the religious person. Dysfunctional religiosity is marked by a strong emphasis on trust, while at the same time the person is deeply untrusting. Trust is an emotional experience of safety in both revealing ourselves and in believing that we are loved and will be treated with respect and compassion. Religiosity is the antithesis of this experience. It sees the love of God as having to be earned through moral rectitude, and by holding onto a set of beliefs even when one cannot integrate such beliefs into one's life. Thus, religiosity is based on fear. The individual who copes with the uncertainties of life through religiosity is a frightened person. This fear often expresses itself through the experience of guilt. Like a child who fears being found out and punished, the individual sees God as a punitive figure, akin to that revealed in the Old Testament, who must be assuaged through penance, or through very painful self-rejection and inner turmoil.

A further irony in all this is that such guilt and fear does not generally make an individual a better human being. I am reminded of Albert Ellis' comment in this regard, that *The more sinful and guilty a person tends to feel, the less chance there is that he will be a happy, healthy or law-abiding citizen ...'* In summary, the picture that emerges when an individual has fallen into the trap of dogmatic and close minded religiosity is one of a very unhappy, judgmental and bitter person, who lives with fear and guilt but cannot find the way to be tender-hearted and forgiving of him or herself or others; this person harbours a wealth of destructive feelings within.

I had a recent encounter with someone who clearly fit this description. I was taking a holiday to Croatia and went to visit Medjugorje as part of the trip. At the airport I encountered a lady who told me she was taking a pilgrimage there. She struck me as utterly devoid of any warmth or having any interest in anything except her upcoming trip. Ironically several days later I attended the mass at the place of pilgrimage only to notice this same person right beside me. She still carried the bitter scowl I had encountered earlier and when during the mass we were encouraged to offer each other a sign of peace, an unfortunate warm-hearted lady reached back to connect with my fellow pilgrim only to be rebutted with a fierce rejection. My angry acquaintance muttered something, and got up and left the church early. I thought," oh my God, can she not see ow unhappy and angry she is, or does she even care?

The roots of this condition are often found in childhood. The person who, as a child, experiences unfair and harsh treatment and who becomes afraid of authority is easy prey to any religious system that allows him or her, as an adult, to repeat this pattern under the guise of truth.

The Abuse of Power

There are many meanings attached to the term power. In the context of this chapter, power refers to our ability to exert influence over the course of our lives. Without some sense of power, we become helpless pawns in the game of life, pushed hither and thither, dominated and used for the ends of other people. I have, for some time, been fascinated by the way that many powerless people become fodder for those who exert a lot of power. Childhood experiences seem to exert a strong influence on a person's way of becoming powerless or powerful. This section is an attempt to describe the essential elements in our approach to power as adults. As such, there are two important elements: powerlessness, and power.

There is nothing so powerless as the helpless child. When that child has been exposed to a destructive environment in his or her formative years, either through direct experience or in witnessing the abuse of loved ones, he or she will develop a damaging relationship to power. One of these outcomes is a continual experience of powerlessness. This sense of powerlessness is revealed in adult life in the following ways: a lack of initiative to solve problems and to create an individual life for oneself; an attraction to people one can depend on for direction; a feeling of being unable to make decisions for oneself; and an inability to leave situations that are hurtful or damaging.

Lack of initiative is rooted in the belief that nothing one does makes any difference. People who perceive themselves in this way feel that life happens to them. They take little responsibility and are often directionless. Instead of developing into adults who have some sense of what they wish to do with their lives, they sit back and let somebody else make decisions for them. This leads to an attraction to people who like to take control. In its initial stages, there is comfort in having someone, or some belief system, to give direction for how to live. Eventually, however, this leads to a growing sense of helplessness.

When people surrender responsibility for their own lives, they risk becoming used and abused. The world is full of such victims, and it is often a harrowing task for those in the helping professions to observe how difficult it is for these victims to break free. Part of this difficulty lies in these people's inability to make decisions for themselves.

Perhaps one of the central elements in having power over one's own life lies in a person's ability to make his or her own decisions. I am continually surprised at the number of people who seem to have lost, or never learned, this ability. Recently, for example, I had a consultation with a woman in her early forties who seems to have little or no sense of her right and responsibility to make decisions for herself. In all the key areas of her life -her marriage, children and job - she has exercised little or no choice, other than to follow what seemed to be the path laid out for her. As a result, she is dis contented about all these areas, and never really felt that she made decisions based on her own needs, ambitions and desires.

During the session we had together, I asked at several points, 'What do you want?' She seemed confused and taken aback by this question, and it became clear to her that she had never asked herself this question while choosing the paths that she did. Thus, she is in a job she doesn't like; in a marriage with someone who is unsuited to her; and had children before she was ready to do so. This is what happens to most people who do not know how to make decisions based on their own needs. They become powerless, and their lives are ruled by externals and the requirements of others.

The third strand of powerlessness is a lack of ability to leave situations that are dangerous and damaging. When people fail to develop a sense of initiative, and combine this with an inability to make personally significant decisions, the way lies open for them to 'arrive' in situations that are emotionally and sometimes physically dangerous. Having 'found' themselves in such a situation, they lack the skill, courage and sometimes the insight necessary to leave. A stereotypical example of this phenomenon is that of an abused woman who is physically brutalised by a pathological husband. Each day she hopes and prays he will change. She tries all kinds of strategies within the relationship to make him become different. Eventually, she exhausts herself and begins to think of leaving. Even when after huge effort she can find some way out, she is likely to return to the relationship. In most such cases, this person has a history of neglect or abusive episodes in her childhood. Her helplessness in that period of her life continues to haunt her as an adult, by removing from her the sense of her own right to avoid needless pain and suffering. This aspect of powerlessness is perhaps the most poignant; some people have died simply because they felt unable to leave the threatening environment.

Power, in itself, is a central element in human life. For any of us to live healthy and fulfilled lives, we must be able to exert some degree of power over our environment. Those who become powerless, as we have seen above, are almost always damaged by the experience. And in many cases, this damage is a direct result of how others misuse power. This section deals with the way that childhood experience can result in a person learning how to abuse power.

The abuse of power is one of the biggest contributors to human suffering in the history of humanity. When we see the abuse of power at a social and political level, we may frown in puzzlement and talk of evil and depravity. The abuse of power is, however, not in essence a political problem (although political change can diminish it by removing or controlling the abuser). It becomes political when the abusive person is elevated into a position where they are visible, and where their abuse is affecting large groups of people. The core element of the abuse of power is neither political nor social - it is in the heart of the individual. Everyone who has become notorious in history as an abusive and destructive human being was that way before they came into public view. And their march to power was strewn in more limited ways with the victims of their abuse.

So we are left with the following questions. What is the nature of the abuse of power? What forces are at work in the abusing person? The answers are manifold, but a central element has to do with the way the abusing person developed and what destructive relation to power lies at the foundation of his being. It is in this realm that childhood experience is of fundamental importance.

There are three essential components required for the abuse of power. These are: a person who is in a position to exert influence over someone; a decision by that person to use this influence in a way that subjugates or damages others; and victims who are powerless to avoid such influence, either because they can see no way out, or because there actually is no way out. When we use this description, it becomes clear that the misuse of power is an everyday and common occurrence.

Some examples that have recently come to my attention help to show its prevalence at all levels of society. The first relates to the misuse of power under the umbrella of religious teaching. A client recently recounted being told by a priest that she could not have a hysterectomy unless her life was in danger. The fact that she suffered heavy bleeding during menstruation and already had more children than she could adequately care for had no significance in the matter. This example reflects an abuse of power. The priest, as a man, had no power over this woman, but in his position as a representative of God and the Church, he could use her beliefs as a lever against her own needs and better judgment. His abuse of this power is reflected in the invasion of her private life and his lack of concern for her health and quality of life. This phenomenon was very prevalent in Ireland during the period when the Catholic Church reigned supreme, and many many women suffered terribly as a result.

This example is useful also in that it highlights the relationship between power and powerlessness. The woman felt powerless because she believed in the absolute authority of the Church. Many others would not have this belief, and would thus not be powerless in this situation. The priest, on the other hand, had his sense of power increased by this woman's submission to his exhortation and control. He, in consequence, became more resolute and convinced of his rightness in the matter, and would have felt more empowered when encountering another, similar, situation. And so the cycle continues

- those in power feed off the powerless, who in turn become more helpless and look more to others to decide their fate.

Many such situations arise on an everyday basis in this and other societies. Examples abound which are less extreme, whilst still often having the effect of changing the course of a person's life. Such instances include the academic professional who marks an individual down in an essay or examination simply out of dislike; the teacher who humiliates a child simply because he or she is having a bad day; the nurse who fails to attend to a patient who is in pain. These are all examples of people who have socially sanctioned power and are wielding it in an unfair way.

Other situations are based simply on physical strength. These include the man who beats up his wife, the mother who abuses her children, or the adolescent who bullies those weaker than him. In the context of this book, we are discussing the person who consistently abuses power out of his or her own unmet needs or emotional distress. In order to understand this problem more clearly, we need to examine what is going on in the interior world of those who need power and who then abuse it.

Many years ago, I began my search for some answers to the nature of human destructive behaviour. This search led me to a serious study of the factors involved in the holocaust. It was of particular interest to me to examine the way that certain human beings behaved when in positions of absolute power, and how others who faced absolute powerlessness coped in that environment. One of the conclusions I reached was that the most dangerous type of person is one who has had an experience of being abused while feeling absolutely powerless and who then is given a position of power. This conclusion is based, in part, on the fact that the worst abuses in that cauldron of evil and cruelty were often carried out by prisoners who had been elevated into positions of relative power.

Psychologists had become intrigued by this reality, and found it occurring in other situations where people were subjected to abusive power. Such instances occurred in prison systems and in hostage situations. Eventually the term 'identification with the aggressor' was coined as a way of describing the way that some people who are exposed to the cruel use of power become cruel when they are given power. What is of great interest to me is that this cycle, whereby the victim becomes the perpetrator, has not been generally accepted as pertaining to the most obvious and common situation where cruel power is combined with complete powerlessness: child abuse.

Powerlessness is an inherent part of early childhood. When a child is abused by those who have power over him or her, they may react to this in adulthood by seeking power. Those who resolutely engage in a striving for power over others are very often trying to compensate for experiences of having had no power at all. Power gives them a feeling of emotional safety; it means that they will no longer experience that terrible feeling of being utterly helpless in the face of humiliation, degradation and violation. When such people then find themselves in a position of power, they are often far more destructive and cruel than those who have not been traumatised by the abuse of power. When they do get into a position where they can wield power over others, the way becomes open for them to act out the anger, frustration and hurt which led them to seek power in the first place.

In order for someone to become cruel in their use of power, they must first be able to detach from any feelings of compassion for their victim. A person who has been abused in childhood has often had his capacity for love and empathy seriously damaged. It is only a short step for him or her to get emotional pleasure and release from making others suffer. I have discussed this process already, under the heading of violence. In relation to power, however, the cruelty to others may not take the form of violence. Rather, it can be cloaked in a garment of social acceptability.

A useful example of this is seen in the raw edge of unregulated capitalism, where power-hungry executives treat those in their employ with derision and ruthlessness. The other major political ideology, that of communism has seen its share of megalomaniacal despots as well. They too wield power with a ruthlessness that is hard to fathom, leaving millions of victims in their wake.

On a much smaller scale there are the very familiar situations that involve the family members of the power abuser. Within the secrecy of the four walls of the family home, the power abuser wields authority with an iron fist. The spouse and children often live in fear and dread of a variety of weapons, such as financial blackmail, emotional and verbal assault and sometimes physical abuse. In so many ways, the power abuser is reliving his own experience as a child, except that in this case he is the perpetrator and those weaker than him are his victims.

Summary

This chapter has examined some of the major outcomes of an emotionally damaging childhood. On reading it, a person might be led to ask 'Can all this destructiveness be a result of experiences that happened in the past?' The answer, in my opinion, is 'Yes'. The long-term effects of a damaged childhood have less to do with a particular series of events and far more to do with the way that human beings build their lives on the basis of experience. When that experience is fraught with fear, loss, trauma, hurt and anger, then the human being who emerges as an adult is seriously affected in the way he or she relates to himself, others and the environment. His or her character is built from the blocks of experience, combined with his or her inborn temperament. The events themselves may be lost in time, but their impact stays alive in the person whose personality has been built around them.

A second question can be asked, namely 'Are these outcomes always a feature of such damaging experiences?' The answer, I believe, is that the degree of injury to an individual depends on the extent to which forces for healing and support were available during the formative years, when other destructive forces were at work. A story related to me by a colleague nicely illustrates this point. As a therapist, he had the occasion to work with a professional man in his mid-forties who had come to him because of marriage difficulties. This man's main problem was an inability to become emotionally close to his wife, even though he loved her very much. It became clear that this problem had its roots in his experience as the child of a violent, alcoholic parent. The emotional confusion and unpredictability of his relationship with his alcoholic mother at an early age caused him to fear intimacy. Although he was able to manage well in other aspects of his life, this problem became more and more intolerable in the marriage relationship. The generally high levels of self-esteem and sense of competency that this man showed in his life intrigued my colleague, as it is unusual for someone who has been reared in such circumstances. It turned out that as a boy this person would work for several hours after school each day with a neighbour. He accompanied this man while he went about his work on a farm. The neighbour was a quiet man who spoke little, but who imbued in the boy a sense of normality and an appreciation of him as a person. This experience stayed with him as he launched himself into the world of adult life

. This story illustrates an important point. Children can and do respond quickly to healing influences. The presence of even one loving and caring adult can make an enormous difference to how the child perceives the world. Alice Miller calls these people 'helping witnesses'. She recounts many situations where children are saved from developing serious psychological problems later in life by the presence of a caring relative or family friend. Not only is this true, but children will actively seek out these people and want to spend time with them. It is as if they have an emotional radar which tells them where they are safe and where they can receive comfort and affection. The people most damaged are those for whom there was nobody.

Certain aspects of the discussion thus far deal with the kinds of human behaviour that is described in terms of good and evil. More specifically, a lot of what has been said can be seen as the presence of evil in human experience. And such evil is real. It is not simply the other side of good; nor is it an outdated religious concept. Evil is the term that we use in describing human behaviour that damages and destroys that which has beauty, value and goodness. Understanding how people can act in such evil ways, towards themselves and others, does not in any way minimise its reality, but it can help us to see a way forward in terms of healing and preventing it. In concluding this chapter, I can do no better than quote Alice Miller, from her book Banished Knowledge: Facing Childhood Injuries:

... evil is real. It is not innate but acquired, and it is never the reverse of good but rather its destroyer. Shakespeare was aware of this. He saw and showed the origins of evil, but never tried to relativize evil by using psychological explanations, as is done in psychoanalysis, for instance. Richard III, Macbeth, and some of his other characters are evil because they are destructive, even when we know why they have become so. Our knowledge cannot alter them. They can change only if they sense, not merely intellectually but with their feelings, how they have been turned into evil people. Only then will they be able to remove the blockages and by experiencing the blocked pain, liberate the abused child who had no wish to harm anyone on coming into the world, the child who wanted to love but found no one to make that possible for him. All he found was barbed wires on all sides, and he believed this to be the world. When he grew up, he built gigantic worlds full of walls and barbed wire, or complicated philosophical and psychological

systems, in the hope and expectation of receiving love in return, the love he never received from his parents when he was an 'unworthy life'. The so-called bad child becomes a bad adult and eventually creates a bad world. The loved child will create a different world, for it is our biological mandate to protect human life, not destroy it.

The next part of the book deals with how we can heal ourselves, and help with healing others, in order to become ready for the true tasks of living a full human life.

Part Three

Healing, Recovery and Growth

CHAPTER 7
Emotional Healing

'The heart has its reasons that reason knows nothing of.'
Pascal

Introduction

At the outset of this book, I discussed the enormity of the task of fundamentally changing the way we live our lives. This section expands and details the elements of such change. Injuries incurred during the formation of ourselves, allied to living for years and sometimes decades using destructive coping strategies, make recovery a complex, difficult but ultimately very satisfying process. We live in a quick-fix culture, in which simplistic notions about human change abound. These influences do little to help people who wish to confront and alter the way that they live. I am going to address this problem here by presenting a model of recovery that I believe takes full account of the intricacies and complexities of human nature.

In this and the following chapters, I will be discussing the themes of healing, recovery and growth. Healing can best be understood as a process (rather than an event), by which something that has been injured or damaged returns to a state of health. Most of us can remember occasions when we fell and skinned our knees. After we picked ourselves up, cried a bit (sometimes!) and brushed ourselves off, something rather miraculous began to happen: the healing process. We did not make ourselves heal, nor had we much power or say in how long it took. The process of healing is built into the nature of living. No surgeon, doctor, or healer makes somebody heal. Rather, they create the best environment for the process of healing to work. I believe this to be true not only for physical healing, but also for healing the emotions. Let's continue the analogy of the skinned knee. Our broken skin healed up in time, but the process could be either hindered or helped by our behaviour. If we cleaned up the wound with antiseptic, then infection was prevented. If we kept the joint inactive, then the scab did not break open. In principle, then, healing is a process that can be helped greatly by our actions and attitude. Much of what I present in these chapters is focused on creating the best of circumstances in which the healing process can begin, or continue.

Recovery has a slightly different nuance in this book. In my opinion, it is an active, intentional process by which a person builds a healthier and more fulfilling life. It might be useful to hyphenate the word (i.e. recovery), meaning to go back over something and make changes to compensate or reclaim loss or damage. In this context, recovery is that period in one's life when significant energy and commitment are spent on understanding and coming to terms with the wounds of the past, undoing destructive patterns and establishing a firm and healthy sense of personal identity.

Many people see recovery as a life-long process. I don't. Based on considerable experience, I see recovery as a special stage in the process of living. In general, this stage, with proper help and direction, takes most people several years, with major change occurring in the first year or two. Naturally, the more severely damaged a person is, the more recovery work needs to be done. It can be said, however, that there is no clear guideline on what direction recovery takes for a person. This is because people can get easily side-tracked (sometimes with the aid of therapy) into cul de sacs that prevent healthy development. Some, for example, can spend years going around in circles trying to sort themselves out, relying on a form of therapy model that might be inappropriate to their recovery needs. Others can spend years with a shopping list of counselling or self-improvement exercises, whilst still others fall prey to a single emphasis on medication to sort out their ills.

In my view, the processes of healing and recovery are based on four pillars: emotional healing; cognitive reconstruction; behavioural change; and spiritual growth. It is interesting to note that psychological and spiritual therapeutic efforts have, during the last three decades, proliferated a vast range of approaches, which tend to isolate any one of these pillars and set it up as the best or only way to recovery. As a result, there is an almost evangelistic zeal associated with certain models.

I do not believe that full emphasis on any one of these areas is a sufficient basis for human development in general, and recovery from formative damage in particular. Rather, the road to recovery is one with different staging posts which emphasize emotional, cognitive, behavioural and spiritual change (not necessarily in that order). All these aspects combine to produce a unique constellation for each individual. It seems important to note that these areas are not as distinct as it may appear. I see each as being akin to the facets of a diamond: no one facet makes the diamond, and no diamond exists without the facets. You may remember my discussion in the introduction to the book concerning the way that, for example, emotional pain can lead to mental anguish and spiritual difficulties may lead to emotional breakdown. The role of each area will depend to some extent on the specific effects of damaging childhood experiences, but it is highly unusual to find that such experiences have not caused problems in all the areas described above. The remainder of this part of the book sets out how each of these pillars of recovery operate. This chapter focuses on the element of emotional healing.

Healing Core Emotions

I am struck by a certain trepidation in beginning this discussion. Part of this has to do with the emphasis that has been placed on the issue of emotional healing in recent times. I have a deep scepticism about many of the trite, and somewhat meaningless, approaches to the emotional aspect of human development that appeared in the 'me' decade of the seventies, and have proliferated since then, particularly in the United States. The enormous growth of the therapy and self-help industry without, it appears, any concomitant change in the mental health of society at large leads me to believe that something fundamental is amiss. Perhaps it has to do with the constitutional right to the 'pursuit of happiness'. James Hillman tells us that "We've had a hundred years of therapy and the world is getting worse".

Or again, perhaps the pioneer mentality that suggests that everything has a solution and will work out if you just do your best, has yet to stand the test of time (the European experience of the last hundred years suggests otherwise). The human condition is more complex than this view allows, and perhaps the field of therapy might do well to take another look at what is meant by the pursuit of happiness.

There are dangers implicit, therefore, in discussing emotional healing. It allows the reader to make a connection between what I say on this issue and some well-intentioned but rather foolish approaches to this topic. As if to confirm my views, I recently had a consultation with a client whose wife has been diagnosed with cancer. His palpable grief and worry for her served to remind me once again that we cannot underestimate the meaning of emotional suffering if we are to give any useful attention to its healing. Having said this, I believe strongly that emotional healing is a central issue in recovery, and I will try to do justice to its intricate and complex nature.

The concept of healing our emotions carries within it the assumption that this aspect of personality can be hurt and damaged. In the earlier sections, I have dealt with the way that this happens, both in terms of the early experiences that cause such hurt and damage, and also how we can become adults who continue to damage ourselves and others as a result. Healing these hurts requires a further discussion of the specific way in which our emotional selves become injured.

Human beings are born with a capacity to react emotionally to external and internal experiences. Thus, the new born infant cries when he feels hungry, cold, or lonely for affection. The physical pain is connected with emotional feelings, expressed in tears or screams. Similarly, when comfortable, warm and feeling safely loved, the infant gurgles and smiles. As the child grows and develops, the relationship between experiences and emotional response becomes more complex. As a consequence of mental development, the child begins to interpret the world. Instead of simply responding emotionally to experience, he or she begins to respond emotionally to the interpretation of the experience. In a healthy, loving and secure environment, the child's emotional responses are generally appropriate to what is going on. His or her interpretation of events is reasonably accurate, and most of the emotional experiences are positive and happy ones.

Conversely, the child who grows up in an emotionally destructive family has experienced ill-treatment, neglect, abandonment and/or abuse. When this happens, the relationship between experience, interpretation and emotional response breaks down and becomes confused. As a consequence, several outcomes to the child's emotional functioning occur that can cause grave difficulty in adulthood. The first layer of damage occurs through the distortion of the primary emotions of fear, anger, love, and sadness.

Fear is an essential emotion. It provides a child with two important tools for survival: an immediate reaction to escape danger; and a need to seek comfort, shelter and security in the arms of a loving adult. When these needs are not met, either through inattention or rejection, a child is forced to live with a sense of danger, and an inability to trust in the help and safety of others.

When during the formation of a person the emotion of fear is distorted, the adult who emerges will develop a distorted relationship to fear. This is reflected in a consistent sense of dread or apprehension; or its converse, which is an inability to avoid danger, leading to self-destructive behaviour. Anger is another essential emotion. In its healthy form, it provides a child with the energy to assert his or her will, and to demand care and respect. It is by nature a problem-solving emotion, which can lead to resolving problems in relationships and a better understanding of the child's needs. A healthy response to childhood anger includes a listening ear and some guidance as to how the energy of the emotion can be expressed in a non-destructive manner. When the emotion of anger is distorted, usually as a result of a hostile reaction of the parent or those in authority, the adult who emerges will have a distorted relationship to anger. They will, on the one hand, be unable to cope with anger in others and as a result be unable to assert themselves ; or on the other hand, will experience rage and engage in destructive behaviour in inappropriate circumstances.

Love is the emotional response to being loved. It is essential in building bonds of trust and affection. In childhood, the healthy response to love is affectionate reassurance and gratitude. When love is distorted, usually through a kind of emotional incest whereby the adult meets his dependency needs through the child, or by rejecting the child's overtures through cold aloofness, the adult who emerges will have a distorted relationship to love. This leads to emotional dependency and passivity, or conversely to an inability to respond with warmth and tenderness to the love of others. Both reactions create great difficulty with intimacy and healthy sexuality.

Sadness is the emotion that helps us to deal with loss, and to recover from it. It is a key emotion in coping with the many losses that being human brings to our lives. A healthy response to a child's sadness includes comfort, letting him or her express sad feelings, and practical help if something can be done to relieve it. A child whose sadness is not cared for in this way becomes an adult who has a distorted relationship with sadness. This shows itself through the chronic sadness of depression, or a hard and cold emotional state where vulnerability is not allowed, either in oneself or in others.

The first layer of emotional damage to human beings is therefore a distortion of any or all of these core emotional states. This distortion is integrated into the person's sense of identity, and several coping strategies are put into place to help the person survive and function. These strategies have been discussed in some detail in the previous chapters. Here I wish to focus on healing these problems. Recovery and growth require that the underlying emotional state be addressed. Two general areas of healing are important in this regard: 1. unblocking feelings that are locked in the unconscious and reveal themselves in nervousness, sadness and physical sickness; and 2. grieving and resolving loss.

Unblocking Feelings

Damaged people are almost always afflicted with trouble in being aware of their feelings. Some walk through life with a very constricted and narrow emotional awareness. Often their bodies carry tense and sometimes painful complaints, while their consciousness of their feelings is almost nil (men are particularly at risk in this area). Others experience only one or two sets of intense feelings, such as sadness, anger or fear. Growing in emotional awareness is an essential part of recovery. Unblocking feelings can be used effectively to help someone to become emotionally aware. By doing so, a person begins to understand his or her emotional make up, and recognises which emotional expressions were allowed and which were disallowed during childhood. Some children, for example, are encouraged to and rewarded for showing sympathy and compassion, often to their distressed parents. As adults, these people will find it relatively easy to experience warmth and tenderness for those who suffer.

These same children could have been punished for expressing frustration or anger. As adults, they will become tense and uptight when they feel angry. The suppression of anger could be so total that the person can no longer identify when he or she feels angry. Similarly, some children are exposed to aggression and are allowed to fight and take out their frustrations on others who are weaker. When they become adults, they may find that the only emotion they can express is rage. When they are hurt, they retaliate; when sad, they knock things or people around; when frightened, they lash out.

These same children may have been ridiculed for showing vulnerability or softness. As adults, they will find themselves getting angry when someone is needy or dependent, instead of being able to express tenderness and compassion. These examples help to show the results of emotional damage on a person's ability to experience and express a wide range of emotions. Such expression is essential for a fulfilled and wholesome experience of life. I have spoken earlier of how a damaged childhood results in a distortion of the core emotional states of fear, anger, love, and sadness. In reclaiming our emotional selves, it is useful to examine each of these emotions and the way we deal with them. By doing so, we can learn to appreciate and savour those emotions that are most injured, and those that prove most difficult to access and integrate into our everyday lives. When this is recognised, much can be done to heal the way we experience and express these feelings.

Perhaps the most dramatic and sometimes dangerous stage of emotional healing occurs when feelings that are frozen within the psyche are brought into consciousness. With those who are very traumatised, this part of recovery needs to be attended to very gently and carefully. A good therapist will be mindful of the dangers inherent in this process. Unfortunately, there are some who see this part of recovery as the only element in healing, and on occasion unlock tremendous pain, fear and anger for the recovering person, in a well-intentioned but clumsy effort to 'get a person in touch with his feelings'. I am particularly cautious about weekend workshops that have this as their focus, when there is no back-up or ongoing counselling to help the individual to integrate and control what is happening emotionally. The encounter group movement (and variants thereof) was - and still is to some extent - particularly dangerous in this regard. Bernard Farrell examines this area very effectively in his play I Do Not Like Thee, Dr Fell; it is a worthy read for anyone contemplating such an approach to emotional healing.

Having set out these warnings, there is still a very important place for becoming aware of, and re-experiencing, blocked emotions. The following are some suggestions that can be used effectively in this regard. Many of these can be integrated into a counselling relationship, a support group, or even with a close friend who is prepared to help with this process. Most damaged people only experience a fraction of their emotional responses; and many, for example, live very functional lives, with a heavy emphasis on logic and practicality. Under the surface, they carry intense emotional energy that is blocked and repressed. They often take the attitude that the past is over and should be forgotten. Others cannot remember most of what happened in their early lives. One of the indicators of repression is a strong negative reaction to the emotionality of others, particularly children. Parents who have strong denial and repression of their feelings cannot cope when their children react with raw emotions. These reactions are often indicators that many emotional reactions have been suppressed and locked away from conscious awareness. Unblocking these feelings requires patience and commitment.

Here I will discuss four major areas that are of value in this part of the process of recovery. Each area has a primary focus of unblocking buried emotions and becoming more emotion ally aware. The areas are: telling one's story; accessing the inner child; creative expression; and body awareness.

Telling One's Story

Telling one's story is a crucial element in discovering one's feelings. A person can begin this process in a counselling setting, in a support group, or alone. The key elements of one's story revolve around the primary relationships within the family. Without knowing our story, we cannot understand how much of what we feel exists as a legacy of the past. I am reminded of Irvin Yalom's comment that damaged people keep trying to make the past into the future. Knowing our story helps us to recognise those elements in our past that continue to trip us up in the present, creating potential problems for the future.

When I refer here to 'our story', I do not mean factual information only. Like all stories, the emotional content is as important as the facts. An example will help to clarify this point. Let us imagine that a man knows he was beaten a lot as a child. This is a fact of his story. The important recovery issue here is how he felt when being beaten. The little child grew frightened and tense, knowing that the parent was going to inflict pain. He flinches and cowers as the first strike hits; inside, his world begins to fall apart, but he tries to maintain some control as the pain washes through his little body. He grows fiercely angry with the big strong adult who does this to him, but cannot express this anger out of fear of further beating. He also feels hurt by the parent whom he loves; he wishes to be forgiven, taken back into fellowship and to become secure in the relationship once again. Damaged people have dozens of such experiences lying undisturbed in their psyche. Telling their stories bring these to light and bring back, for a while, all the feelings that went underground in their effort to cope.

Whilst somewhat reluctant to present 'self-help' exercises in this book, I believe that the ones described below are quite appropriate in relation to improving self-awareness; that is the limit of their focus here. To begin one's story, it is helpful to write out a journal, starting with the earliest memory of both parents. Gradually fill out the details, as they come back to memory, of the nature of each relationship, paying particular attention to the emotional tone of those events that can be remembered. Ask the questions: How did I feel when this happened? What does this tell me about how my mother/father sister/brother saw and felt about me? How did I cope with this event? Continue this chart of events until you have covered all the main events and relationships during childhood and adolescence. Pay attention both to the positive and negative experiences and take time to dwell on each memory, either in joyful reminiscence, or sad and angry reflection. You may be surprised at just how much of those experiences still affects how you live today. As this process continues, much information not presently available to memory begins to surface. If there are very traumatic incidences, such as sexual abuse, this process may not give access to that information. It is, however, a useful beginning.

Accessing the Inner Child

A second element in unblocking feelings is through what is termed inner child work. This is a very powerful technique for recapturing and re-experiencing buried feelings, and needs to be approached carefully. I will describe first the basic rationale of this procedure and how it is viewed today in the therapeutic world. The notion that within us all there is the child we once were is commonly held by many therapists and self-help practitioners. Some call this child the perfect child, or the magical child. For my part, I like to term this the mythical child. There is a good reason for my use of the word mythical. A mythical character refers to a fictional person who embodies truth. Thus, the great Greek mythologies are stories of heroes, heroines, gods, and anti-heroes who carry messages of truth and relevance to the human race. The stories are not factually true, but their themes are. The mythical child within us is the one we discover through our imagination, based on much of what we know of ourselves; it is through formulating a picture of this child that we can discover a great deal about who we are today.

Certain techniques can help to develop a picture of the inner child but, in my opinion, this work is best approached with the help of a trained counsellor in a one-to-one or group setting. Many of these techniques are used in the context of individual counselling, as well as weekend workshops specific ally oriented towards this area of healing. If you choose to deal with this issue in the context of a weekend course or workshop, it is important to have adequate emotional support available in its aftermath.

One powerful technique that can be done alone is the form of writing a letter to your young self. Take a few moments to visualise yourself as a child, perhaps a memory of sitting in your classroom at school, or in bed at night, or out playing. Any memory that comes to mind can provide a snapshot. Then take time to observe yourself as that young child. When that picture is firmly in mind take time to write a letter to that child, telling them what you see in them and how you feel about them. Finish the letter with an expression of love and support.

Creative Expression

A third useful method of recognising lost feelings is through creative expression. I am reminded of Alice Miller's experience in uncovering much of the abuse of her childhood years through the use of painting. Having spent several years undergoing formal psychoanalytical treatment as part of her professional development as a therapist, she began using painting as a form of personal expression. As a consequence, she found in the shadows and hues of her painting many psychological symbols relating to early traumatic experiences. Subsequent to these experiences she became disenchanted with the field of psychoanalysis, and is now regarded as a foremost authority on the traumatic roots of human destructiveness. Her work on interpreting artistic expression in the lives of Picasso, Hitler, Nietzsche and others is indeed fascinating. This example shows us the power that can be unleashed through the use of artistic expression.

The primary areas where our feelings can be accessed through creative expression are music, colours and words. Many people feel that they have no artistic talent, which may be true if we use existing standards of evaluation. The use of creative expression to access emotions says nothing about the artistic merit or otherwise of such expression. It is, in this context, merely a tool to help us get beyond the constraints often imposed by our logical minds and, of course, a person could be nicely surprised to find some hidden talent during this process.

Colours have an immediate connection to feelings. For example, certain colours are said to be warm and others cold; some are luxurious; others are insipid. Marketing strategists and advertising companies use this reality every day in the consumer society. Here we can utilise the same principle to evoke emotional responses and to understand our emotional make up more clearly. A useful starting point is to use poster paints and large sheets of plain paper. Begin by focusing on your feelings and try to express them in colour and shape. Gradually, you will find certain themes beginning to take shape. Avoid interpretation until you are comfortable doing this - let the colours speak for themselves. The very act of expression is providing a channel for your feelings, and this can be relaxing in itself. Furthermore, it utilises right-brain function, often underused among those who have suffered traumatic experiences in early life. Once you get comfortable with this medium, you can begin to draw (either abstractly or representatively) your experiences of childhood events. You might then begin some interpretative work by discussing your creations (disregard their aesthetic quality) with a counsellor or friend. Gregg Furth's book The Secret World of Drawings can be used as an aid in this process.

Music is another very effective way of accessing our feelings. Almost all popular songs, for example, are love songs and the melody lines are what give them the power to touch our heartstrings. My own favourite pieces of music in this regard tell a lot about my emotional make up. Bruch 's violin concerto in D minor, Mahler's 5th Symphony and Tchaikovsky's Pathetique reflect some very characteristic feelings of mine: passion, sensitivity and melancholia. Snow Patrols reworking of Chasing Cars performed at the Royal Albert Hall is sublime. If you are blessed with any musical talent, you can begin to create your own melodies and perhaps write some lyrics. Those of us less gifted have to make do with listening and connecting to the feelings that music can evoke within us. It is important to allow yourself to float into the experience. For many damaged people, this takes practice, because as has been said earlier, the result of emotional damage is a truncating of feelings and a tendency to live only on the surface. Gradually; as you take time to focus on your emotional life, you will find yourself having a much richer experience of your inner world.

Another useful method of accessing feelings is through the written word. One particularly effective technique is letter writing. Most of us think of letter writing as a means of communication with someone else. Letters can, however, be used to help in understanding ourselves and in expressing feelings. For the more literary minded it is worth the effort to read the classic Letters of Abelard to Heloise which tells the story of two 12th-century French scholars and lovers. The tragic ending of their love affair leads both to take religious vows, one entering a convent and the other, a monastery. They reconnect years later through correspondence.

For those less interested in the subject, one glimpse of Army Lieutenant Sullivan Ballou's letter to his wife Sarah before the battle of Bull Run during the American civil war tells its own story.. In the modern world of texting and tweeting we no longer see such gems as *"But, O Sarah, if the dead can come back to this earth, and flit unseen around those they loved, I shall always be near you in the garish day, and the darkest night amidst your happiest scenes and gloomiest hours always, always, and, if the soft breeze fans your cheek, it shall be my breath; or the cool air cools your throbbing temples, it shall be my spirit passing by"* Ballou was killed in battle soon after writing this letter.

Letter writing can be particularly useful in situations where we are unwilling or unable to express these feelings face to face with the person. They may, for example have passed away. In this regard, expressing feelings in the form of a letter can be very helpful. (In most cases, these letters are a private dialogue, and are not sent to the person to whom they are addressed.)

A good starting point is to make a list of all the people who have significantly affected your life for good or ill. This includes each member of your family; it may also include another relative and/or a teacher; in adulthood, it may also include a partner, ex partner or anyone else about whom you have strong residual feelings. Take time to write a letter to each of these people, with particular emphasis on how they have affected your life. Say the things that have gone unsaid; be as passionate as you can, focusing particularly on your feelings. Then try to read this letter to a close friend or counsellor. This will usually result in discharging some of your pent up feelings, which can give great relief. With those relationships that you consider to be over, or that you wish to end, you can slowly tear up the letter and burn the fragments while you imagine letting this person go out of your life.

Writing can be helpful in other ways. One particularly useful technique is that of keeping a journal. This means writing a journal of one's reactions to life experience on a day-to-day basis. This is especially helpful for people who have difficulty in staying in the present, and who are inclined quickly to cut off from their feelings. Journaling courses, usually based on the work of Ira Progoff, are available to assist in developing the skills to use a journal for self-awareness and healing. Those who are blessed with gifts in the use of language can also express themselves through story writing and poetry.

Body Awareness

A fourth major area where feelings can be accessed is through body work. Once again, certain warnings are appropriate in this section. Therapeutic body work is extremely potent in its ability to unlock very deep emotional reactions. It is also a controversial issue within the field of psychotherapy. This controversy involves the discovery that a person's body appears to 'remember' physically traumatic experiences, especially those that occur before the brain has developed the ability to hold images of these experiences in memory. One of the more controversial parts of this area is the issue of birth trauma. Many therapists believe that the body has a memory of birth trauma. Arthur Janov was one of the first to exploit this notion fully (its roots were in the work of Wilhelm Reich); he built a therapeutic intervention programme called primal scream, on this basis alone. More recent approaches are less concerned with the single event of birth, and place more emphasis on using the body's sensations to access a variety of emotional experiences that have lain dormant and out of conscious memory. These methods are particularly useful in helping people who have suffered physical and/or sexual abuse as children.

One of the more popular and well developed - and to my mind effective - approaches is that of Holotropic breath work. Developed by Stanislav Grof, this method uses breathing and music to help a person into an altered state of consciousness where emotional and physical reactions are greatly heightened. The theory behind this method is that unresolved trauma can be released and then integrated and resolved, through the process of re-experiencing and catharsis (i.e. emotional and physical expression). This is, however, only one aspect of the use of breath work; some believe that it is also a very effective means of achieving spiritual insight and transpersonal development.

Other useful techniques are those that focus on the energy field of the body. Several therapeutic approaches have emerged with this as their main function. Perhaps the best known of these are biodynamic therapy, Reiki and SHEN (Specific Human Energy Nexus) therapy. Thus far, these methods appear to be quite successful for some people, particularly when a person cannot respond well to the more cerebral and discursive approach of 'talk therapy'. One note of caution seems appropriate here. These kinds of techniques should be facilitated by a properly trained practitioner, preferably in a peaceful and serene location. Time also needs to be allocated to the aftermath of such intense encounters, so that the person can be debriefed and gradually allowed to return to the ordinary, everyday experience of life. More detailed discussion of the role of therapy is discussed in the section on getting help in Chapter 8.

Grieving and Resolving Loss

Loss is an inevitable part of the process of living. The way that we cope with loss is important in terms of whether we live healthily or stay bound by unhealed wounds. Those who have been emotionally injured in childhood have several areas of loss that may not be resolved. These losses usually comprise the loss of appropriate and healthy love within the family, and the loss of encouragement, affection, guidance and self-worth.

Other losses often result from these experiences. Examples include the loss of a useful education, due to being unable to concentrate on learning; loss of years caught up in the half light of addiction; loss of fulfilment and happiness through destructive co-dependent relationships; loss of a healthy and joyful relationship with one's own children as a result of being an emotionally damaged parent. These, and many others, are the losses that occur during adulthood, often as a direct result of earlier losses in childhood. Coming to realise these losses, and then to come to terms with them, is a very important part of emotional healing.

One of the signs that tell a person that there are unresolved losses in his life is a tendency to live in the past. This is usually marked out by a continuing sense of regret and an ongoing obsession with the question; 'What if?' - 'What if I hadn't dropped out of school?' 'What if I had married someone else?' 'What if I hadn't had children at such a young age?' These and a myriad of others keep us bound by the past, and can prevent us from living fully in the present and planning our lives differently for the future. Grieving loss allows us to confront fully the emotional impact of our losses; in doing so, we can learn from them, let them go and get on with the rest of our lives.

There are several elements in the process of grief. Many of these have been described by people who work with the bereaved. It can be said, however, that grief is not confined to the death of a loved one; rather, it is the human process by which we deal with the loss of anything or person that we have invested ourselves in emotionally. People who were injured emotionally as children are often unable to grieve. This is because the emotional elements of grief were not allowed by parents who themselves were emotionally damaged. The experiences of childhood present many forms of loss; the first day at school, for example, while exciting, also confronts the child with a growing sense that separation from parents is now going to be an everyday reality. When friends move away, there is a loss of their presence and shared companion ship. Then there are the major losses that occur when parents separate, or die.

Even the simplest childish things, however, can be an experience by which a child can learn how to deal with loss - a broken toy, a falling out with a friend, failure in school or in a valued competition - all involve a time of grief. One of the common losses of childhood is the death of a cherished pet, which provides a useful example of how children can grieve in a healthy manner. In a healthy family, such a loss is dealt with in the following way. There is a time of sadness and tearful reminiscence, which is allowed and facilitated. The child is comforted and supported. Then there is some kind of ritual, such as a burial, and perhaps a prayer for the spirit of the animal. In a relatively short period of time, there is usually an attempt to replace the lost pet with a new puppy or kitten. Each of these steps provide a means by which a child integrates the loss, deals with the emotions and becomes free to love again; it also provides a process by which adults can deal with the losses of the past and move on from them. The three elements contained in the above example are: emotional release; ritualising letting go; and replacing the emotional needs that were offered by the one who has been lost. I will deal with each in turn.

Emotional Release

The two major emotional states that come about in the aftermath of loss are pining and anger (shock is not so much an emotional state, but rather a holding operation until the person can let his feelings surface). Pining is an intense longing for that which has been lost. The greater the emotional significance of the loss, the more intense will be the feelings of sadness and longing for its return.

There are many examples of this state in both the human and animal kingdom. When the swan loses its mate, it continues to look for it, sometimes for years. When a cat or dog loses its little ones, it often goes into a state of mourning. A couple of years ago, our cat had her first litter of kittens, whose arrival was greeted with wonder and excitement by the children. Unfortunately, the cat was unable to feed the kittens, due to blocked nipples. We didn't know what was wrong, because we had no experience in the early life of kittenhood. Eventually, the kittens began to die and were too far gone for us to rescue them. This experience had a profound effect on the cat, who moped around, became agitated and searched valiantly for her lost kittens. She eventually became aggressive and spiteful and ran away, never to return. If simple animals can experience such grief, how much more will it play a part in the human response to loss?

Pining is an important stage of the grieving process. It is usually marked out by a period of intense emotional focus on what has been lost. The person becomes very absorbed in his or her feelings, and can easily be seen to be feeling sorry for themselves. For healing to occur, the individual must partake fully in this self-absorbed period. The emotions of sadness, frustration and anger must be allowed to surface and be expressed. It is usually most helpful to do this with the support and comfort of another person. Unfortunately, many people are of the view that feeling sorry for oneself is a bad thing, to be avoided at all costs. As a result, there are a great number of people who have never allowed themselves to grieve over the very real tragedies and losses in their lives. Others remain in a state of shock and denial that such losses have deeply hurt them. The first step, then, in healing loss is to recognise the losses that have occurred, and to access the feelings that go with these losses (much of what I have said in the section on unblocking feelings is applicable in dealing with loss).

A second emotion that often attends confronting losses is anger. There is a sense of 'Why me?', and often a frustrated rage against the person who has left, and/or against life, God and the universe. This anger can be released through physical expression, such as pounding a pillow, competitive sport, using the punch bag at a gym, breaking stones on a beach, as well as some of the other milder techniques described above. If anger from childhood loss is not released, it can easily become an emotional abscess, leading to bitterness and hostility that can last for years and lead to more loss - including the loss of one's health, and the loss of friendship and love of others. This is why it is so important to experience and express the feelings that are attached to the losses of the past. This step leads naturally to the next one, which is that of letting go.

Letting Go

A second stage in grieving for losses involves letting go the emotional attachment to that which has been taken away. Some people never reach this stage, and continue for years in a state of mourning that seems to have no resolution. This is particularly true in some forms of therapeutic situations, where a person begins to realise the full impact of damaging early experiences to their lives. Rather than grieve the losses of love or the terrible effects of abuse in order to get beyond these experiences, the person can find him or herself in a persistent state of self-pity. This often leads to living the life of a victim. There are disastrous consequences for those who get caught in the web of victim behaviour. Everyone around him or her becomes a vehicle through which the sad story can be related. The person becomes totally self-absorbed, and loses any sense of responsibility for his or her own life. Everybody and everything become a source of frustration, and an opportunity for blame. Eventually, people tire of the continual recounting of the damage and injury that has been wrought upon this person. In so doing, they begin to treat him or her as an object of pity, which further confirms to the person that he or she is so damaged that nothing can be done about it.

A recent incident rather humorously describes this syndrome. I was presenting a training course for facilitators who work with therapy groups for adult children of alcoholics. During the presentation, I took some time to deal with how these facilitators could help people to avoid the trap of living lives as victims. I told the story of a client of mine with whom I worked in my early days as a counsellor. One day, this client said that he had some problems with the way the counselling was going. He said it was like I had a bucket in my office, and each week he came in and spent the hour throwing up his emotional state into the bucket. Then, after the session, I empty the bucket and have it ready for the next client. Having told this story, one of the participants caught its meaning and quipped (while drawing an imaginary line across his stomach): 'It's not a scar I have, it's a zip!' In their own dark-humoured way, these individuals captured the syndrome of becoming stuck in the past. While it is essential to recovery to tell one's story, get access to and express the emotions that are associated with its events, it is equally essential to be able to let go, leave it behind and get on with living in a new way.

Letting go sounds simple, but I am continually reminded that this is not so. Again, and again, people delude themselves that the losses are settled and the past is over, while at the same time being consistently tripped up by their unacknowledged connection to it. One very useful way to help in the process of letting go is to perform some kind of ritual which expresses, in a practical way, the choice to let go what has been lost. Several specific forms of ritual can be used. Probably the most powerful of all is that which is an intrinsic part of the Japanese harvest moon celebration. Each year, those who have been bereaved make a lantern which represents the soul of the one who has passed away. These lanterns are then lit and placed in the river to float away into the distance. This ceremony is very evocative and expressive, and can be usefully employed by anyone who wants to break the ties that grief often involves. A small candle can be used to represent each of the losses, and the whole ritual can be shared with a close friend who accompanies you throughout, letting you speak your feelings, shares your silent moments of sorrow and is with you while you say goodbye. When a ritual such as this is used, there can be a sense of relief amidst the sorrow, and a gradual feeling that the ties that have bound you to the past are broken, allowing you to move forward. It is only then that it is realistic to try to replace what has been lost. Another valuable resource in dealing with the grieving process is that of James and Friedman's "The Grief Recovery Handbook".

Replacing that which has been lost

In many situations, people can try to compensate for losses before dealing with the grief involved in these losses. An excellent example is found in what are called rebound relationships. In such relationships, a person tries to deny the feelings of loss through an immediate emotional involvement with someone else. Many such relationships end up in trouble, because the new person cannot replace the one who has gone (either through death or separation). It is important, therefore, in dealing with loss to distinguish between the needs for love that the original relationship provided from the actual person who provided these needs. The desperation, loneliness, and loss of self-esteem that often attend the break-up of a relationship can easily leave a person so vulnerable that he or she reaches out to anyone who shows an interest in them, even if that person is not suited to their real needs for relationship. With this caution in mind, it is still important to try and meet the needs we have that are brought to consciousness out of loss. Human beings are a needy lot! We need a certain amount of love, support, comfort, praise and a lot else if we are to be fulfilled and happy. Much emphasis in modern therapeutic psychology, as well as new age thinking, tends to understate and sometimes even undermine the reality of these needs. The focus of many recovery groups seems to be on making people into rugged individualists who can spurn the need for loving companionship. This emphasis, whilst understandable in terms of helping people to take responsibility for their own lives, and to avoid co-dependency, can have a detrimental effect on individuals, as well as on the community as a whole.

Part of recovering from grief involves replacing that which is lost. If it is a lost love, then a person needs to begin to become available to new friendship rather than pining away in anger and self-pity. If the loss is more practical, such as a loss of educational or career opportunities, then small steps can be taken to plan rebuilding an education or career. Naturally, some compromises may be essential in these areas, and it could take five years to do what originally should have taken two. It can be said, however, that recovery is no small challenge, and one can waste years in regret that could usefully be used to replace the lost opportunities. I explain this to some people by saying 'If you spend another year regretting the past, then next year you'll just have another year in your past to regret.'

One of the more devastating losses a person in recovery faces is the damage that may have occurred in his or her relationships with his or her children. I recently had an opportunity to witness this situation. A woman in her fifties came for counselling because of a family crisis. In our conversations, it became clear to her that she had been injured in her own childhood in such a way that she found it very difficult to experience and express her feelings. One of the results of this was that she had failed to be expressive of her feelings for her children when they were growing up. As a consequence, she was almost completely estranged from her children, one of whom was now in a deep personal crisis.

When she began to see the connection between her way of parenting her child and the crisis he was now in, she became terribly upset. This kind of situation is common among mature adults who begin the process of evaluating their own lives and, terrible though it is, there is a great deal of satisfaction in recognising that new relationships can often be forged with their now adult children. The possibility for love between a parent and a child has no statute of limitation, and there is always an opportunity for healing on both sides. Grieving loss is, therefore, an essential part of recovery. It allows a person to live more freely in the present and to face the future with a positive and life-enhancing attitude.

Summary

In this chapter, I have focused on the importance of dealing with damaged emotions and the specific losses that occur as part of traumatic and damaging childhood experiences. Whilst this kind of healing is a central part of recovery and growth, it is not the whole story. It is also important to learn to cultivate the positive emotions of peace, joy and happiness. These experiences are, however, responses to changing other aspects of one's ways of living. They are in effect by-products of healthier living. By addressing other areas of personal recovery, these emotions begin to flourish, grow and become part of everyday life.

People who have been hurt in their formative years will also find that, as adults, other areas of their personalities have been seriously flawed, and their experience of life has become constricted and often painful. The other principal areas of difficulty are: negative and destructive thinking patterns; futile and inappropriate behaviour; and distorted spirituality. Part of recovery and growth is the process of healing these areas. By doing so, a person can reclaim those parts of being a whole person that were driven underground, or that remain lying like a seed waiting for the warmth of spring before they can begin, tentatively but resolutely, to grow and ultimately blossom. It is to these issues we now turn.

CHAPTER 8
Changing Thinking Patterns

'Do not be conformed to this world but be transformed by the renewing of your mind.'

St Paul

Introduction

A second pillar on which recovery and growth is based concerns changes in the way that we think. You will notice that I am putting an emphasis on 'the way that we think' as distinct from 'what we think'. This is an important distinction. Many counselling approaches that are labelled as cognitive therapy (from the Latin cogito, meaning 'to think') place primary emphasis on what we think rather than the way we think. Popular versions of these approaches span from Norman Vincent Peale's The Power of Positive Thinking through to Louise Hay's The Power is Within You. More scholarly versions are found in the therapies of Albert Ellis (Rational Emotive Therapy) and Aaron Beck (Cognitive Therapy and the Emotional Disorders). All these approaches share a similar view: seeing the human mind as something akin to a complex tape recorder, in which are stored thousands of messages about oneself and the world. The process of change and recovery is to understand these messages, and to change them into ones that assist a person to grow in confidence and self-esteem.

These approaches are worthwhile and have an important role in changing thinking patterns. They are, however, in my opinion insufficient as models of recovery. I believe that they miss an important point, namely that damaged people are affected in the way that they use their minds and not just simply because they have a series of negative thoughts that need to be replaced by positive ones. The human mind is far more than a recording machine. It is actively engaged in filtering information, calculating meanings, interpreting, selecting and rejecting different pieces of information, all with the purpose of developing a view of the world that is consistent and meaningful. These very complex operations of the mind are what become damaged in a destructive childhood experience, setting the person up to operate with less than helpful thinking strategies in adulthood. Recovery, then, means far more than changing a series of thoughts; it means examining the way we mentally deal with experience and it also means restructuring the process of how we think. In order to do this, we need first to examine how destructive childhood experience affects cognitive development.

Damaged Thinking

We have seen in the previous chapter the way that destructive early experience affects emotional well-being. Here we will examine the effects of such experiences on our mental state. A useful tool in helping to understand these issues is provided by one of the foremost cognitive psychologists of the twentieth century, Jean Piaget. According to Piaget, a child does not simply learn a whole series of bits of information. Rather, throughout childhood, as the brain develops the child creates a framework into which his or her experience of the world is put. This mental framework changes gradually, as more and more information is placed within it. Two processes are at work during childhood and into adolescence (and in my opinion, throughout life). These Piaget called assimilation and accommodation.

Assimilation refers to the mental ability to gather or collect information about the world. Let us imagine a child who sees a big red truck arrive at a neighbour's house; the truck has a blue flashing light on top, and the child sees several people all dressed in dark blue clothes and funny hats rush from the truck and begin to pull long red things out of it. Then he sees water being sprayed at the house by men holding the long red things. He recalls a bed-time story read by his mother, and remembers that the people were called firemen. He is now able to collect and assimilate this information into a framework he had for those dressed in these funny clothes. They are firemen.

Accommodation means adjusting something to provide for an experience. Let us imagine this same child a few days later, as he sees a car with a blue flashing light stop outside a supermarket; several men in dark blue clothes get out. He says to his mother 'Look at the firemen'. She replies that they are not firemen, but policemen. The child must now accommodate his framework to take account of this new information. His new framework allows that all men dressed in dark blue clothes getting out of a vehicle with blue flashing lights are not necessarily firemen, but could also be policemen. Further experience then tells him that not all vehicles with blue flashing lights are fire trucks; not all people who get out of these in blue clothes are men; and so on. In other words, his framework for understanding the world broadens and changes in response to more and more experience.

This very simple picture describes the way that children learn to think. Piaget's work is far more complex in terms of how these frameworks operate and how they change through several important stages of development. I am greatly simplifying these processes for the purpose of outlining, in a general way, the fact that thinking is an active and subjective process. In healthy development, there is a gradual growth in the sophistication of the framework with which the person views the world. Old frameworks become obsolete and are replaced by new ones, each reflecting more and more of the complexities in life and the reality that uncertainty is a basic part of life. In damaged children, this process by which thinking develops is stunted, which in turn leads to several destructive cognitive patterns in adulthood.

Destructive Cognitive Patterns

The most powerful determinants of how a child learns to think are the degree to which he or she feels secure in exploring the world and the kinds of experiences he or she is exposed to during the developing years. In a healthy environment, these two elements operating together lead a child to build a reasonably positive and optimistic view of the world, as well as an openness to learn from new experiences. If a child is traumatised in any consistent way, then he or she will develop one of two thinking problems. Firstly, he or she may develop very rigid frameworks that give security, but which do not fit with much of his or her adult experience; and/or secondly, he or she learns to reject or filter out much information that does not fit with his or her framework. The first involves damage to his or her accommodation to new events; the second refers to damage to his or her ability to assimilate information. How do these destructive patterns emerge in adult life?

Every adult experiences life through a set of assumptions about the nature of reality. This is his or her cognitive frame work, and it helps the individual to make sense of and to predict to some extent what is going to happen. Many people are not consciously aware that they hold such frameworks. Rather, they believe that the world is the way it appears rather than that it is, in part, how they have learned to see it. And some people manage never really to test their world view against new experiences.

On the other hand, people who are progressing towards wisdom and maturity are able to let their frameworks change. New experiences are allowed in to broaden the boundaries of their world view. This is a lifetime process for healthy people, because they are not fundamentally afraid of the uncertainties of life; nor are they rigidly adhering to obsolete beliefs because they are afraid of change. This is generally not the case with damaged people. Underlying most damaged peoples' way of seeing the world is a great deal of fear. This fear leads the individual to build what I refer to as defensive world views. These are like mental cocoons which help the individual to make sense of the world without learning anything new. Some of the more common cognitive frameworks are: 1. certainty versus uncertainty; 2. hope versus despair; 3. courage versus avoidance; 4. meaning versus absurdity; 5. guilt versus remorse; and 6. affirmation versus negation.

The process of changing one's thinking involves moving from a destructive and rigid framework towards its polar opposite. All of these have certain emotional correlates, but they are essentially states of mind. Each provides a way of interpreting the events of one's life. The emotional impacts are often directly a consequence of the interpretation. If these emotional aspects are given sole attention whilst the frame of interpretation is ignored, then one is set up for a lifetime of struggle as each event produces a similar emotional impact. When the framework is changed, this has a direct effect on the emotional outcome. This is why similar events can have profoundly different effects on different people. Those with a despairing state of mind, for example, are far more easily crippled by adversity than those with a hopeful outlook.

Certainty versus Uncertainty

A good rule of thumb in this regard is that the more damaged and insecure an individual is, the more he or she will need to be certain that what he or she thinks about the world is true (without continuing to search and explore new possibilities). In other words, his or her lack of internal personal security is compensated for by a sense that he or she knows the 'truth'. Several areas of life can provide this person with a framework where they can find such security. Two are particularly common, and provide useful examples of how this process works. These are religious dogma and political ideology.

Religious dogma is particularly attractive to people who need certainty. They know implicitly that they themselves are not 'big' enough to contain the ultimate truth; knowing also that at a fundamental level they are somewhat powerless, lack all the necessary information and do not have perfect wisdom, they cannot in their own terms claim to know the 'truth'. This produces deep insecurity for those who are fundamentally fearful and cope with their fear by needing certainty. It is helpful to these people if God tells them in some manner or other the 'truth'. They can then claim to know the truth, not on their own terms, but because some being who is big enough to 'know' all the secrets of life and the human condition has told them. Once an individual has become convinced that they have found the answers in the voice of God, speaking through a church leader, a prophet, a Messiah, or through religious writings, then he or she feels much safer living in an uncertain world. A set of explanations and answers becomes available for all that life throws the person's way.

Some religious explanations are far more tolerable and tolerant than others, but essentially each must by definition create a set of people who do not accept the particular set of dogmas and are thus unbelievers. In extreme situations, this group is seen, to a greater or lesser extent, as the location of evil. It is then only a small step to becoming able to justify judging, rejecting and in some cases persecuting those who do not accept the precepts of a particular belief system. It is this process that can make religious belief very dangerous when overlaid on an individual's insecurity. Such religious certitude promotes, in Bertrand Russell's words, *a dogmatic belief that we have knowledge where in fact we have ignorance, and by doing so generates a kind of impertinent insolence towards the universe*. History shows us many examples of just how destructive this process truly is.

Political ideology is also a fertile ground for those who cannot cope with uncertainty. Whilst there are many illustrations of closed thinking among people in this sphere, a particularly useful and contemporaneous example is found in the rise of what is called terrorism. Essentially, in my opinion, those who promulgate terrorist behaviour are for the most part people who cannot accept that the system they attack can have any value, and that their own particular ideology is the right one. Dostoyevsky, long before the rise of European revolutionary terrorism, provides a superb portrait of the justification for terrorist belief and activity. The character of Raskalnikov in Crime and Punishment argues thus: 'The crimes of these people are of course relative and various; mostly, however, they demand... the destruction of the present in the name of a better future. But if for the sake of his idea a man has to step over a corpse, or wade through blood, he is in my opinion absolutely entitled, in accordance with the dictates of his own conscience.'

These examples are rather extreme, but are useful because they show the powerful destructive potential that exists among many peoples' yearning for certainties. Much of the awful destruction to human life and liberty has been promulgated by people who combined emotional pain and damaged thinking with political power. In doing so, they offered those with less power and influence a safe comfort-zone in which to make sense of the world, until, of course, they took away their rights and liberty.

What marks out these damaged people from those who are more balanced in political or religious opinions and beliefs is the degree to which they are unable to take the views of others into consideration. It is their closure to learning or examining the accuracy of their beliefs against new experiences and information that shows a distortion of their cognitive development. There is nothing wrong with having beliefs about ourselves and the nature of the world we live in. But such beliefs need to be accessible to change, to maturing and to rejection. This means that in order to continue growing as a person, none of the beliefs we have about ourselves or the world can be held as being absolutely certain. Living with this reality is, of course, much more frightening for those who were perhaps exposed to chaos on one hand or over-protection on the other during their formative development. In my opinion, however, the realisation that we do not need to be certain of all things in order to live very fulfilled lives can come as a great relief. Furthermore, it allows a person to explore many possibilities that would have been denied in the safe but often arid landscape of dogmatic belief.

Living with Uncertainty

One of the dilemmas intrinsic to the human condition is that people have to live their day-to-day life with the assumptions that their beliefs about reality are true, whilst at the same time realising that many of these beliefs can, and sometimes will, change. In other words, we live our lives continually testing our beliefs against our experiences. When we stop this experimental orientation towards our lives, we stop growing. Some people stop very early in adulthood, resulting in living out boring and mediocrity lives. Others continue to learn and grow gracefully into old age, facing death with even more questions than answers. The irony of all this is that it is these intrepidly curious people who live better and more productive lives than those who failed to confront the reality that life is an experiment in growing and changing.

We cannot, of course, live in a world where we have no guidance from our beliefs, and I am not recommending such a path. I am suggesting that we must continue, in spite of our fears, to confront the reality that we are finite and vulnerable creatures who are very prone to making mistakes of judgment, to settle for less than is possible, and ultimately to fail to mark out our own unique existence on the canvas of life. We must live as if our beliefs are true, whilst at the same time consistently listening to the impact of experience either directly through the events of our own lives or through the opinions of those we respect. The more damaged we are, the less we will be inclined to proceed with life as an experiment. Changing our beliefs from certitude to hypothesis is one of the key elements in promoting an openness to change and growth. A second area of change lies in cultivating hope.

Hope versus Despair

One of the key mental attitudes involved in both recovery and ongoing personal growth is that of hope. We have seen earlier that many people who are damaged during their formative years develop a view of themselves and the world that can be described as hopelessness.

The healing answer to this problem lies in developing hope. In order to clarify the nature of hope, it is worthwhile to distinguish it from something similar that seems to permeate much of the healing profession - naive optimism. Such optimism is reflected in the writings of many self-help authors. It is characterised by the belief that everything that happens to a human being has a reason and is ultimately for the best. Perhaps the most succinct example of this kind of reasoning is found in Scott Peck's book Further Along the Road Less Travelled, where he says 'Now what better news can there be than that we cannot lose, we are bound to win? We are guaranteed winners once we simply realise that everything that happens to us has been designed to teach us what we need to know on our journey.' (In many respects this quotation is not an accurate reflection of much of Peck's writings, but is used here as an example of the kind of belief that abounds in a great deal of self-help literature.)

Proponents of this belief want to help individuals to develop a positive attitude to life and to have an optimistic view of the future. The purpose of this belief is, therefore, to provide a person with a particular type of hope. Here's a gem about illness from the runaway bestseller "The Secret" by Rhonda Byrne. "Our physiology creates disease to give us feedback, to let us know that we have an imbalanced perspective, or we are not being loving or grateful". And, "when a person has manifested a disease in the body temple or some kind of discomfort in their life, can it be turned around through the power of right thinking? Absolutely yes". This form of delusional optimism is, to my mind, essentially dangerous and in the long-term counter-productive to recovery. The view that all suffering has a meaning and purpose for its victim leads to a nihilistic and ultimately deterministic view of the world. This in turn leads to passivity, denial and despair. These outcomes are the direct opposite to what this change in belief is supposed to accomplish. One of the best analysis of this phenomenon is Barbara Erhenreich's excellent book "Smile or Die: How Positive Thinking Fooled the America and Fooled the World."

It is perhaps less well known that this kind of optimistic interpretation of all human events as planned for the greater good is a very old and outdated philosophy which has found a new genesis in modern psychologised society. One of the best critiques of this viewpoint is presented in the novella Candide, written by French philosopher Voltaire in 1769. An important character in the story is an intrepid optimist, Dr Pangloss, who believes that all things are for the best. Pangloss strongly influences the main character, a young nobleman called Candide. The remainder of the story comprises a series of dire and disastrous events, which challenge Candide's acceptance of this sentimental notion. The story itself is hilariously funny in a black way, and is a true satire on what I believe is a very simplistic and silly view of the human condition.

There is no basis in fact for the assertion that many of the experiences wrought on human beings in this world have any reason or purpose for the individuals who suffer them. A child found dying among the corpses in Rwanda and who is nursed back to life has no extra right or claim to life than those whose bodies kept him warm long enough to be found. The adult who squirms in terror as he or she re-experiences the awful trauma of violent sexual abuse visited upon him or her as a child cannot become healthy if encouraged to believe that this happened for some good reason. It is important as a part of developing hope to move in the opposite direction to this kind of thinking. Much of what happens to cause us suffering and pain has no reason in and of itself. When we can accept this, and confront many of the implications for grief and sorrow that come with this realisation, then we can develop a much better and more realistic foundation for hope. Such acceptance paves the way for a mature hope that is not based on denial or a sentimental reinterpretation of the past, but rather one that takes full account of the exigencies and uncertainties of human existence. We do not need to romanticise the past in order to develop a meaningful hope for the future.

What, then, is the nature of this hope? A useful comment from the philosopher Gabriel Marcel provides insight into some of the central elements of mature hope. He suggests that hope is 'nothing but the active struggle against despair'. In this simple phrase, two important facets of hope are recognised. Firstly, it is something active. This means that hope must be cultivated through active attention. It is not simply a cliched belief that things will turn out for the best. Rather, the individual must engage in an active retraining of his or her view of the world, which is often both defeatist and passive. It is the active choice to believe that life can be worth living, that healing is possible and, more fundamentally, that the past does not have to become the future.

Secondly, it is a struggle. Cultivating hope for damaged people is sometimes painful and taxing. The easier road is for them to give up and to slide into a vortex of depression and bitterness. It is sometimes surprising to people like myself in the caring professions to witness just how deeply entrenched people can become in insisting that their helpless and hopeless view of life is the reality. To struggle against this belief is often very painful, for it means that many of the secondary gains, such as self-pity and the sympathy of others, must be forfeit. The struggle involves doing battle with one's belief that giving up is best, that it's all too much to bear, and that what we make of our lives is of no significance.

Hope is, therefore, by its nature not so much an answer to a specific set of circumstances. It is rather an orientation of a person's mind or intellect toward the future, a future that does not exist, but has yet to be created. And the nature of that future will, to a significant degree, be influenced by the stance a person takes toward his or her own self-determination and belief in healing, recovery and growth. The key beliefs, then, that need to be cultivated are: that healing the wounds of the past is possible (often with the help of others); and that our dreams (or at least some approximation of them) can come true, if we set ourselves about the work required to make this possible. One of the necessary steps in realising such hope is that of developing courage.

Courage versus Avoidance

Closely related to the concept of hope is that of courage. I remember attending a conference a number of years ago where I engaged in an interesting debate with two colleagues on the subject of courage. I had asked the question 'What it is that differentiates people who survive and grow towards healing and fulfilment from those who do not?' My friends were of the view that hope was a significant element in this process, whereas I cast my vote on courage as a major influence. As the discussion continued, we began to move toward the position that hope and courage are intrinsically related. In order to be courageous, one must have some hope, whereas hope without courage is sentimental and does not lead a person to engage in the struggle to overcome adversity. Rather, it just leaves them wishing for change and optimistic that some outside agency will come to their rescue. Courage without hope can lead to a very self-destructive way of life. Thus, whilst courage is a central element in changing one's life, it needs to be based on some sense of hope that such change is both possible and worthwhile. What, then, is the nature of courage? Once again, it may help to examine what it is not. Many people see courage as a sort of hard-headed, fearless orientation. Whilst there are many people who appear able to approach life in a bullish and domineering manner, this does not make them courageous. A story about an episode that occurred during the First World War, recounted by Victor Frankl in the book Psychotherapy and Existentialism, nicely illustrates this point. *A Jewish military doctor in the Austrian army was sitting next to a colonel when heavy shooting began. Teasingly, the colonel said: 'Just another proof that the Aryan race is superior to the Semitic one! You are afraid, aren't you?' 'Sure, I'm afraid,' was the doctor's answer. 'But who is superior? If you, dear colonel, were as afraid as I am, you would have run away a long time ago.'* Frankl goes on to comment that 'Fear and anxiety as such do not count. What matters is our attitude towards facts rather than the facts themselves. This also applies to the facts of our inner life.'

So here is the crux of courage: it is always expressed in the presence of fear and not in its absence. If we are not afraid of something, then it takes no courage to address ourselves to it. This is why some of the most frightened people in the world are also among the most courageous. These are people who choose, in spite of their fear, to confront that which they fear. I meet these kinds of people regularly in my work as a counsellor. What is of particular interest is the general trend among courageous people initially to expect that counselling will help rid them of fear before they have to confront that which is causing the fear. Having made the initial courageous step of asking for help and being prepared to admit to their fears and struggles, they expect that the counsellor or therapist has some magic potion that will ease or get rid of their pain. It is often with disappointment that they learn that such magic potions do not exist (or those that do are more destructive in the long term), and so they are left with the reality that over coming fear means going through the experience of fear and out the other side.

Courage, therefore, is particularly important in the process of healing and recovery. This is so because people who have been hurt and damaged during their formative years are more fearful and vulnerable than others. This is true even among those who cover their fear with aggression and violence. The strength and destructiveness of their reactions are in proportion to the level of fear being masked by these reactions. One might well ask 'What is this fear all about? and 'Why should such people be more fearful?' Ultimately, the answers to these question lie in two directions. The first concerns fear of loss; the second is fear of emotional and/or physical pain.

Fear of loss is often extreme in damaged people. They have a more fragile sense of their worth and sense of safety in the world than others. In turn, they often attach their need for safety and their sense of value to things outside themselves, such as a relationship, a good job, a big car and so on. Anything that threatens the person's attachments causes a major emotional reaction, which is essentially grounded in fear. This is because the loss of such attachments has a meaning far above the value of the object itself. It is the perceived loss of self-worth that produces such reactions. In order to recover and get beyond such a fragile state, these people need to confront their fear and learn to experience loss of their attachments with grace and acceptance. In so doing, they begin to undo the crippling effects of having externalised their self-worth.

The second area where fear plays a central role is the fear of being hurt. A useful analogy in this regard is that of physical damage. When a person has been physically injured, their healing process leaves a scar. This scar tissue is neither as strong nor as supple as healthy tissue. As a result, it is more vulnerable to further injury. For example, any woman who has given birth through caesarean section will be aware that during a subsequent pregnancy there is a danger that the tissue from the initial surgery may rip while under the pressure of a second labour.

People who are emotionally damaged carry around an equivalent emotional scar tissue, which leaves them more sensitive to feeling very hurt in situations that an undamaged person would cope with more easily. Those, for example, who feel rejected react with powerful emotions to a new rejection. Some become so fearful of rejection that they will not take the risk of becoming close to another person. The level of pain felt in a new rejection is so great, because it is wounding the person in a place where they are already seriously hurt. It is of fundamental importance to becoming a healthy person to understand that many events in the present carry the possibility of great pain because of unhealed wounds from the past. Otherwise, the levels of emotional reaction seem inappropriate and to make no sense to the individual reacting to the event or to those close to him. Maria's story helps to clarify this point.

Maria and Tom have been married for several years. Tom is a successful business man, who has only recently begun to understand his own emotional make up. Maria is a highly intuitive person, with a deep connection to her feelings. They both attend a social evening that has an important business element. Tom spends most of the evening circulating with clients and potential clients, leaving Maria pretty much to fend for herself in the company of another couple. As the evening continues, Maria becomes more and more agitated, angry and sullen. By the end of the evening, she is deeply hurt and enraged. Tom has no understanding of this reaction. Days later, Maria is still reacting and no amount of apologising on Tom's part can ease her anger. Whilst Tom is blameworthy for being insensitive, Maria's reaction is extreme and seems like an overreaction. In discussion with Maria, it became clear that her reactions to the situation were related to her experiences as a child.

The most important man in her life, her father, consistently neglected her. She was never made to feel special, and all the landmark events of childhood such as birthdays, first Holy Communion, first days at new schools, examinations and the time of examination results were marked out by his lack of interest and support. This wound left her highly susceptible to being badly hurt in situations where she felt neglected. Her reaction to this feeling was also a replica of the past. She quietly withdrew in a helpless anger, unable to take control of the situation and express her feelings and ask for what she needed.

Courage in this situation required choosing to confront the situation, despite the risk of feeling more hurt. And this is perhaps the key element of courage: it is the choice to put oneself in the situation where there is a risk either of loss or hurt. Of course, there needs to be some discretion used in deciding which situations are worthy of such risk. A useful guide in making such choices lies in knowing those situations where the goal is worthy of the risk and where there is some chance of it working out to one's advantage. It is not courageous for a person to walk unprotected through a ghetto at night: it is stupid. The choice to be courageous must have some meaningful purpose in terms of one's growth toward becoming a healthy person.

There are two useful elements in developing courage. One is the encouragement and support of those who care. Most adults remember the role of encouragement in helping them as children to take some risks with fear. Simple events such as going to the dentist, walking past a fierce looking dog, or even learning to get back up on a bicycle after a fall. The friendly encouragement of a parent or other loving adult can be recalled as giving the impetus needed to take the step. And it became easier next time. As adults, we are no different in our need for encouragement, whether it comes from our partners, friends or a professional helper.

A second helpful approach in developing courage involves breaking down feared situations into manageable steps, each requiring some courage, but not producing intolerable fear. Practicing this approach focuses one's mental energy on solving difficult situations rather than avoiding them. These are the intellectual steps that precede the actual doing. Such an approach results in changes in the mental framework that facilitates a healthier way of living. The key beliefs in regard to courage, then, are that it is not about being unafraid - it is in choosing to confront one's fear. Such confrontation must, however, be guided and directed by some meaning and purpose. This leads on to the fourth area of changing mental attitudes, that of finding meaning in adversity.

Meaning versus Absurdity

It is important, as part of a healthy and recovery focused mental framework to find meaning and value in experiences that were hurtful and damaging. From the discussion above, you may have been left with the impression that suffering, toil and pain are meaningless and ultimately absurd. This does not have to be the case. The experience of adversity allows people to express some of the highest qualities of human life. In this sense, all suffering can have meaning. However, this meaning is not built into any particular experience; nor is it a meaning which exists in advance of the experience. Let us take the example of one of the most traumatic experiences - that of the death of a child. Can anyone really believe, in good conscience, that the death of one's child is a useful, necessary, or purposeful event? I have worked with many people who have had their lives seriously damaged by such an experience. Despite the need for some to believe that their child is in a better place, most are left with the anguished question of why such an event had happened to them. And, of course there is no answer - except the one which says there is no answer.

I remember watching a film called Grand Canyon, which to some extent deals with the question of why terrible events happen to some people. The main character, a wealthy white man, finds himself lost in a dangerous ghetto when his car breaks down. He is approached by a group of young African American gang members. These rather vicious thugs begin to threaten his life, and he is saved by the arrival of another African-American, a salvage truck driver. Friendship develops between these two men. One of the significant moments in the film occurs when the white man asks his saviour why such an event should have occurred where he almost lost his life. His friend's answer is interesting.

He compares much of what happens to people to a situation where someone is attacked by a shark near a crowded beach. The shark has no personal vendetta against the particular individual; the person is not chosen for any particular reason- he just happened to be in the wrong place at the wrong time. It could just as easily have been someone else. This view reflects the reality that most human suffering has no meaning in and of itself. This seems to be true even within families where children are abused by their parents. The child had no choice in being born to such parents. He or she finds themselves in that family. The abuse would probably occur to any child who happened to exist in that situation. It is, therefore, rather futile to search for meaning for many of the events that cause suffering by asking the question "Why did this happen to me?'

Where, then, lies the meaning and value of such experience? The answer, in my view, lies after the fact. Certain people are set apart from others by the way that they deal with suffering. Some develop a numb stoicism that leaves them detached from their feelings and distant from other people. Others become embittered, jealous, spiritual wrecks. Still others rage and punish others for their plight. Amongst these reactions one finds a set of people who have coped differently with their experience. These are people who in some way seem to have become better people, more generous and understanding of others, whilst continuing to grow and become richer in mind and spirit.

What is it that sets these people apart? We cannot argue that their pain was any less severe, or that they started out from a better place. I believe that such people have been able to harvest something good from the wreckage of their traumatic experience. It is this process of searching for something good to take from any experience, no matter how difficult or painful, that allows people to get beyond the anger, bitterness, and pessimism that afflicts so many of those who have been badly treated in life. And so we reach a different conclusion than those who say that all things that happen to us have meaning. Rather, we can say that it is a defining characteristic of human beings to be able to find value in events that cause pain and suffering. The potential for meaning lies within the person, and not within the event.

There are a myriad of stories to which I could refer to illustrate this point, but one in particular comes to mind. It is probably because the person in question tends to quote me on occasion. Toward the end of a consultation with him, I said: 'Well Peter, Believe it or not it might be fortunate that you became an addict, or you would never have recovered!' This kind of statement may seem quite odd, yet I truly meant it. Peter, a professional man with all the trappings of success, had become addicted to a powerful prescription drug during his forties. He almost ruined his career as well as his health. Fortunately, his family intervened and he responded by going for in-patient treatment. What ensued was the most painful and traumatic period of his adult life. During his treatment, it became clear that prior to his addiction he had managed to isolate himself almost completely from any kind of real human contact. He lived in a fantasy world, and used money to solve all problems, including the care of his relationship with his spouse and children.

It was only a short step for him to begin using drugs to fill the 'hole in his soul'. Within a relatively short period, he was a drug addict. His addiction produced the crisis that led him to change. This change (as with recovery from most forms of addiction) involved dealing not just with the addiction, but also with the plethora of destructive life patterns in which he was engaged. The process was slow and painful, but ultimately well worth the struggle. Did his becoming a drug addict have meaning? The answer for Peter is that it had, but it could just as easily have killed him. Its meaning lies in what he chose to do about it. Perhaps a different kind of crisis could have led to the same outcome. Drug addiction in itself is of no value and is very destructive. Peter was able to learn profound lessons from the experience, and for the first time come to terms with his life and work at living it differently.

Seventy years ago, Elizabeth Kubler Ross set out four stages by which people cope with the reality of death. Since then, many writers have applied these stages of denial, anger, bargaining and acceptance to other human tragedies. I believe that a fifth stage, whereby a person finds some value in traumatic experiences, helps people to move on in life with hope and courage. Furthermore, searching for something of value, such as a lesson learned, a broader outlook, a greater sensitivity to others, a better understanding of oneself, can also come about by applying this process not just to the events that happen to us, but also to our own mistakes. This leads to a crucial fifth element in changing our mental framework, namely turning guilt into remorse.

Guilt versus Remorse

You may be somewhat surprised to see the issue of guilt being addressed in a chapter on thinking. Most people think of guilt as a feeling, and would expect it to be dealt with in the previous chapter. Guilt, however, is more complex than a single emotional feeling, and in my opinion is very strongly influenced by the way a person interprets an event. And this interpretation belongs firmly in the realm of thinking. Guilt is a special form of anxiety, which occurs once we believe we have done something that is wrong in terms of what we hold as the right and good way to behave. It has a very important function in the human story. As such, it is something which can be useful in helping people to live better lives, or it can be distorted and have very destructive effects. In damaged people, guilt is distorted in two ways. Firstly, and more commonly, guilt can be present to a very high degree, causing much unhappiness and pain. Secondly, some people experience too little guilt, leading them to be able to carry out very destructive and sometimes inhuman behaviour with little or no internal emotional sanctions.

Excessive Guilt

Guilt is only useful if it helps us to avoid repeating a mistake, or encourages us to become better people. It operates within a human being in the following way. Every person has some mental picture of the way he or she should be. This is called the ego ideal. When a person does something that contravenes this ideal, he or she experiences an uncomfortable feeling, which is called guilt. It is, in essence, a form of anxiety related to the person's failure to meet his or her expectations. For a healthy person, these expectations are realistic and can change with maturity - the level of anxiety experienced is in proportion to the level of failure. Some people, however, are crippled by the presence of guilt in their lives. They feel guilty about almost everything - guilty for what they feel, for what they think and for what they do. Underlying this experience lies a lack of love and respect for themselves, and a desperate need to be perfect in all things, in order to feel accepted. In most cases, this extreme level of guilt has grown out of a childhood where there was little forgiveness and genuine mistakes were punished as wrong doing. In order to reverse this tendency, these individuals need to change their mental framework, from demanding perfectionism to one of recognition of weakness and self-acceptance. These steps involve two crucial elements in making a realistic evaluation of one's activities: responsibility and control.

Responsibility

Many people who are devastated by deep feelings of guilt have accepted responsibility for things that are outside their control. Responsibility carries within it the concept of choice. If we did not choose a certain course of action, then we are not guilty of it. Thus, the myriad of thoughts that can cross our minds from time to time are not within our control and cannot be considered to be our responsibility. This is a crucial piece of information for those who are haunted by destructive thoughts, which occur without their intention, and often cause painful feelings of guilt. Sometimes there are reasons - such as suppressed anger - for the appearance of these thoughts, and it is important that these underlying causes are discovered and resolved (the anxiety condition of OCD is however a different matter and the often-horrible intrusive thoughts are not a result of unresolved or unconscious motives). It can be said, however, that those who are afflicted in this way need to accept that they are not intending nor trying to create such thoughts; furthermore, by dwelling on them, they often increase in magnitude, causing more worry and concern. It does little good to obsess on them; a better way forward is to accept that they occur, but that they will not in themselves cause anything bad to happen.

Another area where people who suffer from excess guilt are afflicted is by experiencing certain destructive feelings or unacceptable desires. Once again, these can cause a lot of worry and heartache, and only increase in magnitude when the person focuses too much attention on them. Feelings come and go in the ordinary hum of life. They are like the wind gusting to and for outside the person's control. Seeing them in this way can relieve guilt and lead to greater acceptance, which in turn reduces the claim these feelings can have on a person's emotional and mental energy. Destructive or undesired feelings that occur regularly only sometimes carry an important message to the individual, and it is important that their source be isolated and resolved. In themselves, however, they need to be seen just for what they are: uninvited visitors that need to be recognised in passing and then let go. Such thoughts or feelings most often do not lead a person to do anything destructive, and this is where the issue of control comes into play.

Control

Turning guilt into remorse centres on the issue of control. Remorse refers to guilt feelings that occur in response to what we do, as distinct from happenings that are outside our control. At some point, a person can make a choice to turn destructive thoughts and feelings into some kind of action. If that action is destructive, then the person is responsible for its occurrence. When that happens, he or she becomes guilty of the event. For those who suffer from an excess of guilt, it is important that they use this as a guideline to help them make a realistic appraisal of the events surrounded by their guilt feelings. If by appraising a situation in this manner they come to the realisation that they have acted in a way that is offensive to their own values, then they have experienced real guilt as distinct from what is called 'neurotic guilt', and they need to address it in a way that leads to healing. Two areas for such healing are forgiveness and making amends. I will discuss these in some detail in Chapter 10.

A Lack of Appropriate Guilt

Some people emerge into adult life with a capacity to engage in very destructive behaviour, such as using people without any concern for their welfare, or hurting people, treating them badly, beating or abusing their children, committing crimes with little or no feelings of guilt. Many people who have experienced active addiction to a substance such as alcohol also engage in these kinds of activities during the course of their addiction. Lack of guilt for these activities is often underpinned by the person's failure to experience an emotional link to those who are being hurt. There is little sense of empathy for the feelings of others, a lack of compassion and a lack of value for the rights of others. These elements are often grounded in the individual's early development, where the capacity to feel for the experiences of other people is laid down in early relationships. When we hurt those with whom we have emotional bonds, we feel guilt; if we do not develop these bonds, then we can, to a greater or lesser extent, treat people badly with impunity.

A second and related strand to lack of guilt lies in the way some people can isolate their feelings for others into certain compartments, allowing those outside their boundaries to be treated differently. Useful evidence for this process is provided when we examine how ordinary young men and women are trained to kill others in warfare. In order to train successfully such people to kill others, the enemy must be portrayed as essentially different and inferior to the kinds of people the soldier identifies with or loves. The enemy becomes a gook, a slant eye, a nobody - then he is easier to torture, maim or kill. Similarly, whole groups of people such as blacks, Jews and Muslims have been identified during certain periods in history as different and inferior to those who persecuted them.

Lack of guilt, then, is related to what we believe about people whom we mistreat. These beliefs may be underpinned by destructive emotional energy, such as repressed anger and hostility; they allow justification for acting out such anger whilst avoiding feelings of guilt. When the emotional forces that underlie these beliefs have been addressed, then the beliefs have no further function. It is then that the individual's true unresolved issues that led to destructive behaviour come to light and, in general, a healthy experience of remorse will ensue. Whether a person is overly sensitive to guilt or finds that its absence has led to grave destruction, the recovering individual needs to use his or her remorse in ways that heal - insofar as it is possible - the damage wrought upon him or herself and on others. Some guidelines about how this can be approached are presented in Chapter 10.

Affirmation versus Negation

Affirmations are positive and encouraging statements that are practiced in order to supplant the many hundreds of negative automatic thoughts that often, unconsciously, cause loss of confidence and self-hatred among damaged people. Much has been already written elsewhere on the topic of using affirmations in changing thinking patterns, and many self-help books are available to enable people to proceed with this venture.

While it is neither useful nor necessary to repeat the content of such books here, there are, however, some aspects regarding the use of affirmations that require discussion. The first can be stated in the form of a question. From whence do such affirmations come? In the main, they are devised by counsellors and therapists working with a particular idea of the nature of a human being. Thus, affirmations such as: 'I have everything I need to become a beautiful person'; 'I am getting better every day'; 'I am divinely inspired to choose the right partner' are to a large extent based on a middle- to upper-class WASP (White Anglo Saxon Protestant) model of the ideal person'. They are also influenced by a romantic vision of damaged people. Not all damaged people are broken down, sorrowful and lacking in confidence and self-esteem. Some are arrogant, brutal and sometimes evil. What affirmations can be used by a poverty stricken, orphaned Puerto Rican, or for that matter an overworked, burnt-out partner of a chronic alcoholic. Or by someone who abuses those around him.

The difficulty I am raising here is not with the concept of using affirmations, but rather their source. Such affirmations are devised to replace negative self-statements that were learned through exposure to others. But these new affirmations are also second-hand, generally devised by someone who has no knowledge of the particular individual who is going to use them. I don't believe that a list of somewhat sentimental exhortations is appropriate to the needs of most people in recovery. Rather, affirmations in my view need to have two qualities to have any sustainable value: they must be true; and they must be relevant to the particular individual. Some examples may help to clarify this view.

Let us take the scenario of a successful executive, who manipulative and ruthless behind a facade of charm. He stands in front of the mirror each day, and affirms himself by saying 'I have all I need in my power today to succeed in my ambitions'. Then he goes out into his world of business and lies, manipulates and blackmails people into buying products that they don't need and perhaps cannot afford. Here is an example of an affirmation that is true and works for this individual. The problem with it is that it is being used by the sick part of the person to keep him sick. It is therefore inappropriate. The affirmation this man could better use is one which says 'Today I have everything I need in my power to practice honesty and integrity'. But who is going to tell him, and even if they did, what would motivate him to listen?

Let us imagine also the scenario of a depressed woman whose children, into whom she poured her life, have grown up and left home. She wakes up beside her alcoholic husband, who smells of sweat and stale booze, a scenario that has gone on for as long as she can remember. She thinks of the telephone being cut off that day and the letters from the bank. She stands in front of the mirror and looks at the wrinkled face and the hollow eyes looking back and affirms herself by saying 'I have all I need right now to have a bright and happy day'. Here is an affirmation that is appropriate (having a bright and happy day would be really good for her), but it is not true. In the scenario I have in mind this person needs a lot of help, support and hard therapeutic work in order to access what she needs in order to be a fulfilled person.

The great limitation of using affirmations devised by others is that it is so easy to choose ones that are either untrue, or inappropriate. A much better source of affirmations lies within the individual. More specifically, I believe that within each of us there is a motivation to love and be loved; often in very damaged people this is just a whisper from their subconscious, and yet it is there. This element in the human psyche can be accessed as a source of the particular affirmations that will stimulate and encourage growth. Moreover, the kind of affirmations one needs to use will change in time as growth continues. It is often useful, either by means of counselling or support groups, to check with others the truth and appropriateness of an affirmation that an individual wishes to practice. This approach has the benefit of tailoring the affirmations being used to the particular recovery and developmental needs of any given individual. It avoids the culture bias in a lot of what is written on the subject and leads, in my opinion, to a far more effective way of changing one's thinking.

Summary

This chapter has examined some of the key elements involved in the second area of recovery and growth, namely changing one's pattern of thinking. Its focus has been concerned primarily with the mental framework through which we view and interpret the experiences of life. For most people who have been subjected to trauma or neglect during formative years, these frameworks are often negative, limiting and sometimes destructive. By becoming aware, and understanding the role of such frameworks, a person can begin to make the changes necessary for a healthier and more productive life. The next chapter concerns itself with a third major element of recovery, that of changing what we actually do.

CHAPTER 9
Changing Behaviour

'Man becomes truly human only at the moment of decision'
Paul Tillich

Introduction

Thus far, I have discussed healing the emotional wounds of the past as well as developing a healthy thinking framework. These are crucial steps in the process of recovery, but they will bear little fruit if not attended by changes in the things we do and the way we do them. Changes in behaviour are fundamental to becoming a healthy person. In my opinion, it is what people actually do that reveals to what extent they are on the road of recovery and growth. This chapter examines some of the more important areas where change needs to occur. To follow some of the recommendations herein will require much of the courage I discussed in the previous chapter; others may be greeted with anticipation and relief, a surprising realisation that some elements of growing up can be joyful and easy. In my experience, most recovery involves changes in five key areas: 1. getting help; 2. having fun; 3. building healthy relationships; 4. re-evaluating one's career; 5. caring for one's body.

Getting Help

The previous two chapters have outlined some of the major issues involved in setting out on the road of recovery. It is not always possible - nor is it to be recommended - that these changes be attempted alone. The first part, then, of changing behaviour is often the decision to seek help. In general, there are four broad areas where such help is available: professional counselling and therapy; non-professional support groups, including twelve-step fellowships; medication; and residential treatment. To help clarify what might be most appropriate or suitable to different needs and experiences, I will briefly out line the strengths and weaknesses - as I perceive them - in relation to each area of help.

Counselling/Therapy

I have combined the areas of counselling and therapy for the sake of brevity, and because these two areas overlap to a significant degree. Counselling is generally considered to be a brief form of therapy, which is directed toward specific and identifiable problems. Therapy is usually considered to be concerned with deeper, less obvious, problem areas and occurs over a longer term.

Until recently, there has been a stigma attached to the notion that a person might need to seek the help of counselling/therapy in order to resolve personal problems. This stigma grew out of the belief that to experience difficulties in one's personal life was akin to some kind of mental condition; to be less than normal, to be weak and perhaps somewhat crazy. Underlying this stigma is the belief that people should be able to sort out their own lives without help. This is of course untrue. In every culture known to man, there have been members of the community whose elected position was that of healer. The pastoral work of priests, rabbis and elders are western equivalents of the healing role of shamans, medicine men and witch-doctors in other societies. In modern western societies, this healing role has also become the territory of counsellors and therapists.

Given the economic principles of western societies, the role of healer has become a profession which is to a large extent unsupported by the state and therefore many people have to pay for these services. For some people, this poses a real difficulty, not just in financial terms, but also in terms of the principles involved. As one client put it to me: 'I can't help but be cynical about, and feel somewhat humiliated by, the fact that the only real conversation I have in my week is with someone I pay.' I hold the view that people who have consultations with me pay for my time, for the educational element involved in therapy, but they do not pay for the quality of the relationship, because this is not something that can be bought. I think Jeffery Masson 's book Against Therapy has much useful insight into this matter of the dangers inherent in the role of healing as a professional career.

What, then, is the value of therapy/counselling? To a very large extent, the answer to this question lies in the quality of any such counselling and its suitability at a particular time for any particular individual. Research shows that counselling has a chequered history in relation to its effectiveness. This is partly due to the enormous proliferation of ideas about what is involved in the process. One book on my shelves outlines over 250 types of therapy from, believe it or not, 'cooking therapy' through to 'soap opera therapy'. Given such a mish mash of ideas as to what comprises professional help, it is perhaps worthwhile to suggest some of the basic requirements that appear to mark out effective counselling.

A counselling relationship is usually built up over a number of months, and sometimes years. My own beliefs and experience lead me to the view that effective counselling and therapy has certain crucial core elements. These can be divided into two categories: those that are characteristic of the climate of the relationship; and those that belong to the process of what is actually done in the time spent with the counsellor.

The Climate of the Counselling Relationship

The climate of an effective counselling relationship refers to the feelings that are experienced during the encounter. Because every person is different in personality, it seems more appropriate to describe the characteristics of the climate of the relationship rather than the personality character of the counsellor. One kind of person may be more easily able to create the right atmosphere for a client than another, and no amount of training or experience will guarantee that a counsellor will be able to do this with all potential clients. A simple example of this reality is found when we realise that some clients are far more at ease with a female counsellor, whereas others prefer to do their work with a man. When undertaking the process of counselling, it is important to look for the following elements in the counselling relationship: safety, trust, warmth and respect. These, to my mind, are essential ingredients and require brief explanation.

Safety refers to the gradual sense that the counsellor will not further hurt you, reject you, or attack you. For many people in the initial stages of counselling, this sense of safety is both crucial and difficult to develop. Having had a lifetime of covering up their vulnerability, it is extremely difficult for them to reveal themselves. They are often afraid that if they become truly known then they will be abandoned and rejected. Counsellors work hard at trying to establish this sense of safety, because without it the healing process is bound to fail. It is important to recognise that if such a feeling does not develop, this does not mean that the counsellor is incompetent; it may merely be a matter of incompatibility between the two people. And to some extent there is no point in flogging a dead horse in this regard. If after a period of time there is no indication that a sense of safety is developing, the person may need to seek help elsewhere.

A similar story exists in relation to trust. Whilst safety and trust are similar in nature, trust is, I believe, a broader concept. Within the context of counselling, trust refers to the belief that the counsellor is going to see you through whatever crises occur. It is also a sense of confidence in his or her understanding of what is happening to you. Sometimes during the experiences of counselling, a person feels that he or she is going to fall apart at the seams. It is especially important at these times that there is a sense that the counsellor has seen this happen before, and that he or she will be a source of strength and support; and furthermore, that he or she will help the person negotiate the currents and rapids to get to safer ground.

Warmth and friendliness are also essential ingredients in effective counselling. I remember vividly having a conversation with a professional counsellor during my student days. Towards the end of the discussion, as I got up to leave, this person looked at her diary and commented 'Oh God, not this awful man.' I looked at her and said 'I hope that is not a client you' re talking about.' She blushed deeply and changed the subject. I was rather horrified by this incident. In my youthful naivete, I assumed that counsellors would not perceive clients in this way. In the years since then, I've learned that counsellors - myself included - have their biases, likes and dislikes, just like any other human being. We as a group, however, tend to be more tolerant, understanding and interested in people than, say, a group of accountants, insurance salesmen or orthopaedic surgeons. There are times, though, when, there is some difficulty developing a friendly atmosphere between counsellor and client - as with any two people. Sometimes this is due to what is called transference. This occurs when either party reminds the other of someone who has hurt them in the past. Another possibility is that of projection. This occurs when one party sees in the other an aspect of personality that they dislike (often unconsciously) in themselves.

It is useful to examine these within the counselling situation, as they sometimes provide a rich seam of emotional energy that has gone underground. If after examining such possibilities it is still difficult for either party to establish a friendly interaction, then it is better to go elsewhere. One of the advantages of paying for a counselling service is that the client can more easily decide to choose someone suitable for his or her needs. On rare occasions, there are people who cannot be friendly with anyone, usually because of a hostile, bitter orientation to the world. But just because a person doesn't particularly like one particular counsellor does not mean that it is because of a personality problem.

A fourth element involved in the climate of the relationship is that of respect. One can feel safe, trusting and friendly with out necessarily believing that one is respected. Respect in the context of a counselling relationship is based on the notion of equality. This might be summarised as the belief that both the counsellor and client are made of the same stuff. Neither is intrinsically better than the other. This is often a difficult hurdle to surmount, because for the most part the relationship starts off on an unequal footing. The client often puts himself in a somewhat subservient position, and is likely in many cases to idealise the counsellor. This is an understandable element of the early stages of the relationship. In time, however, a gradual change needs to occur, whereby both people see each other as equals, jointly engaged in a task. I like to envisage this as being akin to a psychological and spiritual journey. The counsellor joins the client at a certain point along his path in life. Together, they explore the terrain and utilise the counsellor's understanding of some aspects of the pitfalls, danger zones and necessary difficult climbs, but at all times it is the client's journey that is central to the communication. At a certain point, they reach a clearing and part company, the client having learned some new navigation aids, having matured and been enriched by the time spent with his guide and companion.

When we look at counselling in this way, we take it from the realm of a 'sick' person being treated by an 'expert'. Rather, we see it as a much more respectful and equal relationship. It is a gift and a privilege for any counsellor to be engaged at this level in the life of another human being and it is important for any person considering entering a counselling relationship to evaluate the kind of person they will privilege with this gift. This does not mean, however, that counsellors are simply good companions in the voyage of exploring one's life. They must be this at least, but there are some special things they offer; these are the elements of what actually happens in the relationship.

The Process of Counselling

During the 1960s and 1970s, there was an explosion of interest in counselling, most particularly in the United States. This interest then came to our shores and is exemplified by a proliferation of all kinds of counselling courses. Some focus on particular theories and equip the student with specialised techniques to apply to the counselling process. Others emphasise a broad spectrum of viewpoints and practical aids. Still others are designed for application to specific types of problem areas such as stress, addiction, or sexual dysfunction. In my opinion, effective counselling has at least four aspects: educational; clarifying; directional; and empowering. In discussing these, it is important to keep in mind what I have written above in relation to the context in which these processes occur. The nature of the relationship is as important as these particular processes in terms of healing, recovery and growth.

The Educational Aspect

I am using the term educational here in its broadest sense, namely that a person who goes through a process of counselling learns a great deal about himself, and also about human development and personality formation. Thus, for example, a person who seeks counselling for stress problems related to overwork may need to learn about how people become workaholics. She may need to learn about how the need for achievement becomes paramount if it is used as the only way that she can begin to feel like she is a worthwhile person. She may explore how these messages were communicated to her in her family and at school. This information may be given verbally by a counsellor, or through suggested reading of useful material. Naturally, a person who seeks to avoid responsibility, is lazy and indolent will not need the same information as the overworking, over-responsible, burnt-out workaholic. Rather, he may need to explore the ways that he learned to suppress anger, to choose not to try rather than risk failure, and so on.

Another part of the educational aspect lies in getting to know and understand parts of oneself that are unconscious. Joseph Campbell, in his book The Hero with a Thousand Faces, describes beautifully the importance of this process. In his view:

The unconscious sends all sorts of vapours, odd beings, terrors and deluding images up into the mind - whether in dream, broad daylight, or insanity: for the human kingdom, beneath the floor of the comparatively neat little dwelling that we call our consciousness, goes down into unsuspected Aladdin's caves. There not only jewels but dangerous jinn abide: the inconvenient or resisted psychological powers that we have not thought or dared to integrate into our lives. They are fiendishly fascinating too, for they carry keys that open the whole realm of the desired and the feared adventure of the discovery of the self.

A variety of techniques are available to counsellors in this regard, ranging from analysis of dreams to art work, guided imagery, etc. These are used to open up areas of personality that have been denied, repressed or just ignored. Long-term counselling and therapy make most use of these approaches, because the goal of counselling of this nature has less to do with solving a particular problem and more to do with the client reaching a deeper insight into him or herself.

The Clarifying Aspect

Most people who engage the services of a counsellor are confused. Some are completely mixed up and at odds with themselves; others are, to a greater or lesser extent, in a state of disarray. Confusion is one of the great gifts of life, for it is the prologue to change. Show me a person who has never been confused and I will show you someone who has never learned anything of value. Confusion that doesn't resolve into some learning and change is, however, chronically distressing. The counselling process assists a person to become clearer as to the nature of his or her confusion and to get to a place of clarity around it. Part of a counsellor's role is to help in this task. In this, the counsellor acts much like a tracker following a trail. By attending to non-verbal signals, asking perceptive questions, following associations, feelings and contradictions that seem to make up such confusion, the counsellor gives the individual an opportunity to discover the roots of his or her difficulty, and hopefully the chance to make better decisions based on more accurate information.

It is important here to mention that counselling can also bring about great confusion, especially in its early stages. This happens when a person realises that many of his or her life decisions were the result of factors that no longer are important, or healthy. Central elements of one's life like ones relationships and career have often been based on such decisions and therefore come under scrutiny, which may lead to fear, insecurity and confusion. Thus, things can often get worse before they get better. And although this is often the case during the counselling process, the need to explore and clarify these matters is essential if a positive outcome is to occur.

The Directional Aspect

One of the great illusions in the field of counselling relates to the notion of non-directive counselling. All useful counselling is directive, in the sense that it has a direction. Some counsellors give clear account of the direction in which a client is guided; others, because they assume the mantle of non-direction, often don't know the direction. When people speak of non-directive counselling, they mean that the counsellor is not going to tell the client what to do. Rather, they are going to help the client 'make up his own mind'. Any psychologist worth his or her salt knows that this view is trite and simplistic. Making up your own mind through a counselling process is like asking a person to choose any colour he likes as long as it's either blue or yellow. The 'mind' a person is 'making up' has already been heavily influenced by the process of counselling. And this influence is central to the function of counselling.

Take, for example, a simple case of a man who is very dissatisfied with his boss. He comes for counselling because he is afraid on the one hand of losing his job, and on the other he wishes to quit. At this point he is confused, upset and only sees a choice of two options. Effective counselling in this situation would explore other possibilities. The individual may be reacting to his boss because he has a general problem with authority figures; then again, the boss may be acting unacceptably, or it may be a matter of a personality clash. By exploring these issues, the person gains an understanding of what is actually happening in his work relationship. When some understanding of the elements of the problem is reached, the counselling task moves towards finding effective strategies for dealing with it. In this example, several options could be explored - assertiveness training, undoing fear of authority, stress management and the like. This example is one of the simpler tasks that occur in a counselling situation, yet the whole process has had a direction from the beginning.

Another, and more subtle, area of the direction that is implicit in even the most non-directive counselling is the impact of the values of the counsellor. Clients, in general, look up to the counsellor and become aware rather quickly the he or she has certain views and opinions about how life should be lived. Regardless of how the counsellor tries to hide these from the client, they are at work in the counselling situation. It is essential that the counsellor recognise his or her preferences and comes to terms with them. This is why counsellor training puts such an emphasis on counsellors' self-knowledge. Otherwise, the client may be subtly directed by values of which neither the counsellor nor the client is aware. In taking on a process of counselling, it is useful to check with the counsellor how he or she views a healthy person, and the outcome that he or she is going to pursue jointly with the client. One helpful way to do this is to discuss the particular type of training that the counsellor has had, as well as the kind of problem areas with which he or she is most familiar.

Related to this issue is a trend that developed during the 90's and evolved into a serious controversy within the field of counselling. This controversy concerns what is termed the false memory syndrome. (A lucid and rather frightening picture of this phenomenon is presented in the book Making Monsters, by Richard Ofshe.) The essential element of the controversy was that some therapists convinced their clients that they had been sexually abused as children when, in fact they hadn't. Furthermore, using techniques such as hypnotism, visualisation and other suggestive methods the therapists created and implanted memories that were not real. These well-intentioned therapists were so convinced of the rampant presence of sexual abuse within the culture (particularly in the United States) that they saw it at every juncture, and end up convincing their clients in this regard. The awful outcome from this social contagion was not only that people were led to believe that they were abused, in some cases they went on the accuse wholly innocent people, sometimes their parents, many of whom had their lives destroyed as a consequence.

The other side of the argument is that sexual abuse was, and perhaps still is, a rampant force within society and is only now emerging as a result of the therapeutic climate whereby it is safe to bring these repressed memories into the light. In addition, any casting of doubt on the uses of therapy in discovering the extent and depth of sexual abuse is considered to be a form of denial, and perhaps a conspiracy to assist and enable the abuse. Whatever the outcome of this debate, it has shown that counsellors and therapists have very significant powers of influence where their clients are concerned. And it behoves potential clients to retain their independence and critical faculties when engaged in the process of counselling.

The Empowering Aspect

I have already discussed some aspects of the topic of power in an earlier chapter. Here, I wish to comment briefly on the way that counselling helps people to experience more power in their lives. Many clients who engage the services of a counsellor have, to a greater or lesser extent, lost control of their lives. This may be due to damaged elements in their personality, which are reflected in becoming trapped in destructive relationships; and/or becoming caught up in compulsive or addictive behaviour. In other cases, the loss of power may be a generalised experience of no longer feeling that one has the strength to make choices for one's own welfare.

It may seem paradoxical that the directional aspect of counselling is almost always focused on the person becoming more powerful. Counsellors assist in this process through encouragement and support, often combined with specific suggestions regarding effective ways to solve problems and to build up one's emotional strength and resilience. The opposite to empowering is dependency. It is one of the pitfalls sometimes encountered in a counselling relationship, whereby the person becomes over-dependent on the counsellor. This trend is widespread in the United States: where dependence on one's 'analyst' for even the simplest decisions is almost an institution. I believe that this is a grave error, and is probably related to the financial and commercial reality that counselling and therapy is now an industry. Cultivating dependency for financial gain is a travesty, especially when the stated aim of such an industry is to help people become free and healthy individuals in their own right. This in no way rejects the notion that dependency is sometimes an essential stage along the way to growth, but it is only a stage; any effective counsellor should be gradually working with a client towards independence, both in the therapeutic relationship and in all the other significant relationships in his or her life.

The above is a rather brief sketch of what to my mind are core elements of effective counselling. My hope is that it will be a useful guide to help any reader who engages in counselling to make some critical evaluation of what is best for him or her in this regard. It may also help to evaluate the effectiveness of any help being sought. Another area where people can benefit greatly is through support groups and twelve-step programmes.

Support Groups and Twelve-Step Programmes

One of the most significant developments in the areas of healing and recovery began in the 1930s, with the evolution of what is widely known as the twelve-step programme of Alcoholics Anonymous. This programme was developed over a period of years by two individuals, both alcoholics -a businessman named Bill Wilson and a doctor called Bob Smith. In their joint search for a way toward recovery from alcoholism, they devised a programme based on their own experiences, and incorporating the spiritual psychology of Carl Jung, the writings of philosopher/educationalist William James, as well as the influence of the then current Christian evangelistic renewal known as the Oxford movement. In the decades since then, the programme has developed and proliferated. It is now used as a basic model of recovery for a wide variety of areas of human suffering, most of which have strong addictive or compulsive characteristics; these include gambling, drug addiction, eating disorders and relationship difficulties (particularly those concerned with relationships with addicts of one sort or another).

Twelve-step programmes have been enormously beneficial, and to date have helped hundreds of thousands of people find a way back to sobriety and health. On closer analysis, there are several reasons for the success of this model. Those who partake regularly in the programme experience three fundamental influences, outlined below. (For a more thorough analysis of addiction see my book: "Understanding Addiction: A common Sense Approach")

Firstly, the programme is acknowledged as spiritual in nature, and the first step is concerned with the individual's recognition and acceptance that he has become powerless over a substance or activity. The term addiction comes from the Latin *addicere*, which means 'to give oneself up, or over'. Addiction occurs when a person gives himself up, or over, to the addictive substance or activity; it then takes control of his life and eventually destroys him if he does not find recovery. The twelve-step programme acknowledges this, and provides the possibility for the individual to supplant the activity by giving himself up or over to something else - a higher power, and to the programme itself. This can have a remarkably healing power.

A second strand in the effectiveness of these programmes is that of fellowship. The recovering individual is influenced and supported by the fellowship of others in a similar situation as himself. The encouragement and, more crucially, the sense of identification found among fellow members, give a very positive basis for continuing sobriety. Added to this is the influence of what is called sponsorship, whereby an individual with a long period of sobriety takes the role of sponsor or mentor with a newly recovering addict. The healthy example provided, as well as advice and support, has often stopped a new member from returning to his addiction in moments of crisis.

Thirdly, a change of environment and lifestyle (crucial elements in recovering from addiction) are made possible by partaking in the programme. Most addicts have consistent and habitual ways of acting out their addiction. Frequenting particular pubs or betting shops and the company of a set of equally sick companions make it very difficult for them to cease their addiction. Being part of a fellowship provides new avenues to friendship and different recreational patterns, the bowling alley and coffee mornings replacing the card table and the pub.

Twelve-step programmes have some limitations. In ge neral,it can be said that when an addiction grows out of the pain of a damaged and hurt person, the programme - whilst providing much by way of helping that person stay sober and learn a new way of living - will not be able to address his deeper needs for healing. Rather, the person may stay away from his primary addiction only to find himself addicted to something new, perhaps including an addiction to the fellowship itself! This is evidenced in the numbers who spend decades in the fellowship, but seem to go around in circles, continually telling the same old stories and showing little in the quality of their lives that suggests they are really getting any better.

The positive effects from 12 step programmes for dealing with alcoholism has led to it now being applied to a plethora of other problems not confined to the area of addiction. The ACA adult children of alcoholics for example uses the twelve-step model but in a different way. Other examples are CODA Co-dependents Anonymous, SA Sex Anonymous OA Overeaters Anonymous, GA Gamblers Anonymous to mention a few of the more well-known support groups using the 12-step model.

For a significant number of recovering addicts, much of the damage to their personalities will have been covered up through addiction and is often out of conscious awareness. It may take some period in counselling, combined with continued involvement in the fellowship, to get beyond the cycle of being stuck at a particular place of being dry, or clean, but not sober and healthy.

Other Types of Support Groups

Not all support groups use a twelve-step recovery model. Many, such as those concerned with specific issues like depression, bereavement, mental handicap, etc., provide information and discussion facilities. These group meetings are often very useful in giving people an opportunity to meet others who struggle with similar problems or life events, and to learn more about how to cope with them. Information about their availability can usually be accessed through a health information centre, citizens' advice bureau or through the local doctor.

Residential Care

Two specific areas of residential care are common. Short stay (four to six weeks) residential treatment programmes for addiction, and hospitalisation under psychiatric care for emotional disorders.

Residential treatment for addiction has become very common in recent decades. The most common model used in this approach is termed the Minnesota Model, which combines the twelve-step programme with other forms of counselling and group therapy. These programmes are, in general, privately run commercial concerns offering a wide range of professional intervention. It is scientifically impossible to assess (once a person engages in either form of recovery) if treatment centres are any more successful than the twelve-step programme on its own.

One of the major differences between the voluntary fellowship approach and that of a treatment centre lies in that with the former those concerned for the addict can access help through these agencies and learn how to deal with the addict differently so as to encourage him or her to enter treatment. This means that the addict may get into recovery faster than if left to 'bottom out' and join a programme of his or her own accord.

Treatment centres vary in their success rates, and anyone close to the issue of addiction realises that there will be a percentage of addicts who will not recover, no matter what happens to them. The decision to undertake treatment for addiction at a treatment centre is a difficult one for many people. In general, if after trying through a twelve-step programme and on the advice of professionals familiar with the problem of addiction, an individual is unable to abstain from or control her habit, then it may be the best option.

The strengths of good residential treatment complement that of the twelve-step programme in the following ways. It takes the person out of the familiar environment and provides him or her with a drug- or activity-free context in which to take stock of life. It provides support and identification through the other members of the treatment group. It provides counselling and education that help speed up self-understanding and, most importantly, it provides weekly after-care group meetings once the individual has successfully completed the residential period of treatment.

Some weaknesses have come to light in the residential treatment model. Firstly, like private counselling, it often has a commercial element, which means that there are financial constraints on who can afford it. Secondly, because it is an intensive and relatively short-term treatment, there is a tendency to apply the model to everyone, as if each addict was not a unique individual whose addiction has its own unique story and reason for its existence. Two aspects of treatment have come in for questioning in this regard. The first concerns the role of denial. It is a reality that most people who suffer from addiction are in denial and require 'help' in order to break through their defences. Heretofore, in a zeal to accomplish this task, there have been numerous situations where the confrontation of the addict has taken such a form that many suffered unnecessarily. In some cases, these people have needed help to heal the wounds visited upon them by over-zealous practitioners, who mistook the addiction for the person and lost sight of the fact that some addicts are the most sensitive and gentle people in the world. Thankfully, there is a gradual turning away from these over-confrontational approaches to those in addiction, and a greater recognition that it is the person and not the addiction that is being treated.

Hospitalisation

In general, certain people are recommended for residential care in a psychiatric hospital or in the psychiatric unit of a general hospital because they can no longer cope with day-to day living. In most cases, this decision is taken by a doctor or psychiatrist, and it is considered by them to be in the best interests of the patient. One of the primary concerns of these practitioners is whether or not the individual is posing a threat to his own life, or that of others. Hospital care is therefore reserved for the most severe cases of emotional and mental disorder. The principle of giving true 'asylum' to people in such states is a good idea, but the history of such care leaves much to be desired.

We have much to learn about the facilities that will encourage a person to find his feet again after serious emotional collapse. The institutional care that is available at present requires continual improvement, both in terms of the training that is given to the people most involved with those in distress - namely psychiatric nurses - as well as a more considered approach to the main elements of this kind of treatment, the use of medication. At present, it is preferable for most individuals to avoid a hospital setting, if at all possible. The dangers implicit in institutionalizing people are now recognised (albeit more for financial reasons) by those with responsibility for health care, and we are witnessing a focus on returning people to the 'community' (whatever that is) much more speedily than in the past. In general, a stay in a psychiatric unit might provide a person with time and space to collect himself and strengthen his ability to return to some kind of normal functioning. That is about the limit of its function at present and, in not a few cases, even this is difficult to achieve.

Medication

The use of drugs for the treatment of emotional problems has, at times, become a controversial issue in the fields of psychology and psychiatry. This area is likely to become even more controversial, as a result of recent developments in psychopharmacology (the science of brain chemistry and the effects of certain drugs on its functioning). In general, many who work in the field of counselling psychology and psychotherapy see a limited use for certain types of medication as a part of treatment, whereas those in the field of psychiatry place a heavier and, in some cases almost exclusive, emphasis on drug treatment. Any book which attempts a comprehensive examination of the issues involved in healing damaged emotions must address the use of medication. In order for a person to make a knowledgeable decision about whether or not to use medication, three categories of information are required: what certain drugs actually do; the potential or actual addictive properties of these drugs; and their potential, or actual, side-effects.

Before examining these areas, there is a further question that underlies different approaches to the use of drug treatment, concerning the causes and symptoms of mental and emotional disorder.

One side of the argument (the psychiatric approach) suggests that emotional distress and thinking disorders are in general caused by changes in the chemical functioning of the brain, and therefore are rectified when the brain is treated chemically in order to restore the balance. In this view, drugs are seen as treating the cause of the disorder. The second view suggests that changes in brain chemistry are often a result of emotional damage and faulty thinking, based on destructive learning experiences. Drugs that are used to chemically re balance the brain are therefore treating the symptoms; not only are they failing to deal with the underlying causes, but in some instances they have the effect of making a person unable to gain insight into what is wrong at the root level of his or her psychological functioning. An added complication exists between these two views, in that a change in brain chemistry may continue even if the initial cause is isolated and dealt with. It is probably apparent to the reader that this book takes the second approach.

These differing views contain large philosophical questions about the nature of the human being, ones which cannot be explored fully here. In essence, these questions concern whether or not we use our brain, and as a result affect its functioning, or whether our brain uses us and determines our functioning. The answer lies, perhaps, somewhere in between. One strong piece of evidence which supports the view held here is found, ironically, in the recent experiments within the pharmaceutical field. These experiments are used to help develop new generation of drugs that are being lauded as revolutionary in the treatment of mental distress, and will be discussed in more detail below.

The experiments use a new, very refined, high technology brain scanning method called positron emission tomography (PET). By asking people to focus on certain activities or subjects, changes in brain chemistry are recognised, sad thoughts affecting one part, and pleasurable thoughts another. In terms of drug development, it is then the task of the scientist to synthesise substances that affect these different parts in order to 'treat' the appearance of symptoms.

If we look closely at this approach, we find that when a person focuses on certain thoughts or experiences, his or her brain reacts in a certain way. It only a short logical step to see that what people think about, or are familiar with, affects their brain chemistry. Damaged people -as we have seen in the early part of this book - have much destructive and negative experience on which to focus. This (on the basis of the research discussed above) will affect their brain functioning. Thus, life experience affects our chemical balance. Drugs which attempt to 're-balance' the brain without attending to the underlying perceptions, memories and experiences that have produced these changes cause a split between what the brain state is signalling about our lives on one hand, and the emotions we are experiencing on the other.

This split between our experienced emotions on the one hand and the way we have been affected by, and learned how to cope with life on the other, is potentially dangerous. For centuries, people have attempted to produce 'good feelings' without paying attention to the reasons for having bad feelings (sometimes with some horrific consequences). I see no real difference (except in terms of safety, which has yet to be proven) between the recent developments in chemical treatments and older formulae (those that include all kinds of drugs, including alcohol) in this regard. A very useful comment on this subject comes from Stephen Rose, an expert on memory at the Open University, cited in the New Scientist as follows: 'Think of aspirin; it solves the problem of toothache, but it would be silly to argue that toothache is caused by lack of aspirin.' Taking this metaphor, a bit further, we can see the disastrous consequences of treating toothache over a long period of time with aspirin, or any other painkiller for that matter. Eventually, infection could set in, causing grave physical disorder. The optimism, and at times almost messianic fervour, that is greeting the advent of the new pharmaceutical potions may yet prove premature. One of the more trenchant critiques of psychology in general and the growing reliance on psychotropic medication is that of Theodore Dalrymple's "Admirable Evasions. How Psychology Undermines Morality"

A second question relating to the role of chemical treatments for those in emotional distress in modern society are the economic issues that surround their care and treatment. I remember several years ago having a discussion with an economist on the subject of health care; at one point, he said that when it came down to practical reality, a choice had to be made between the number of hip replacements that could be made for the price of a major organ transplant. This kind of pragmatism also invades and informs the treatment of those who are emotionally and mentally distressed. What does one say to the thousands of individuals who attend their local doctor complaining of anxiety-related disorders, often crying out just to have someone listen to them? Or to those who are disadvantaged, lost or alone in a society that provides little by way of human tenderness or opportunities to seek and find peaceful surroundings in the company of people who care? It is far easier and less expensive (in the short term) to think of these people as having something organically wrong with them (with no substantial evidence in the majority of cases), and to select from the cornucopia of drugs available one which will alleviate some of their suffering without ever addressing the fundamental problems that cause this suffering. The recent epidemic in terms of such suffering is now recognised as the problem of loneliness, which research shows is now killing as many people as heart attacks and strokes.

A third major issue.in relation to the use of drugs in treating emotional distress has its roots in the gradual takeover of science as a way of learning about life and the human condition. In medicine, the primary emphasis is on viewing the human body as a highly sophisticated physical machine, run by an even more highly sophisticated chemical and electrical apparatus called the brain. Using this approach, medical scientists have made vast inroads into the treatment of disease and disability. It was only a short step in logic to believe that the success of medical treatment for the body could be repeated in attempting to 'cure' what became considered diseases of the mind and the emotions. After a century of trying, there is little evidence to show that treating mental disorder by physical means has had much success either in clarifying biological causes of these disorders, or in curing them. What success has been achieved appears to be mainly in developing treatments that alleviate symptoms through various types of action on brain function. This, to my mind, has a very narrow but sometimes useful place in the treatment of distressed emotional states.

The reader is probably aware by now that I am rather cautious about the use of this kind of medication. The difficulty I encounter is that, on the one hand, people should not have to suffer the awful experiences of being psychologically overwhelmed; while on the other hand, the reality is that these drugs do not cure anything. in the long term. I believe that the minimal use of such chemical intervention should be married to a comprehensive healing approach to the individual's distress.

Getting help is important in the process of recovery. This section has briefly examined the core areas where such help is available. It is important to note that people who use the help of others who treat their distress in a humane and informed manner can greatly enhance the process of healing and recovery. Furthermore, it is a real step in the right direction to acknowledge that receiving such help is no stigma, and it is often a far better path to take than a stubborn and resolute commitment to going the road of healing alone. A second crucial element in changing behaviour is learning to have fun.

Having Fun

Several years ago, I read a critique of self-help psychology called Psychological Seduction: The Failure of Modern Psychology, by William Kirk Kilpatrick. I was most impressed by his argument that people who are involved in recovery groups or in individual therapy take themselves too seriously. It is always a risk that those of us who' endeavour to discover who we are and how our lives have been shaped and influenced by our formative experiences will forget how to have fun. We can so easily become obsessed with ourselves, continually searching each experience for some new level of understanding. Eventually we become boring people, using self-help jargon and psychological clichés in every conversation. Recovery becomes a serious and grave undertaking, rather than a joyful and life-enhancing process. Of course, recovery has its painful and sorrowful times, but if it is real it must also have the effect of freeing us from the chains of our past and helping us to become expressive and playful people. Having fun means learning what every undamaged child knows: how to play. As adults, there are three strands that are useful in reclaiming this important part of living. These are: avoiding unnecessary suffering; cultivating a sense of humour; and sharing in adult recreation.

Avoiding Unnecessary Suffering

The key phrase in the discussion here is that of unnecessary suffering. I agree with Scott Peck in his belief that growing and changing often involves suffering, and that it is the avoidance of necessary suffering that often leads to stagnation and despair. There are those, of course, who avoid any kind of suffering at all costs, and who often end up suffering greatly- and causing others to suffer as a result. However, there are a significant number of damaged people who are afflicted with an attraction to misery, and it continues to amaze me how easily such people make life tough for themselves. This tendency shows itself in the simplest everyday experiences, such as not paying attention to their needs for proper food and rest, having continued contact with those who hurt them, taking on tasks with which they are unable to cope, and so on. Having never learned how to know what they need and how to pursue it, they can only identify with those aspects of life that are hard and sorrowful. It's almost as if some people have an internal rule of thumb that says 'Why do it the easy way when you can do it the hard way'; or similarly 'If it doesn't hurt, then it's meaningless'. To emotionally intact people, this seems a crazy way to live. And, of course, it is.

An example from my own life might clarify this point. When the film Schindler's List came to the local cinema and a friend of mine invited me to go along to watch it. I declined the offer. During my twenties, I spent several years learning what I could about the holocaust as part of a study which I undertook concerning the psychology of guilt. I read, widely and tried to cover most everything of significance that had been written about the holocaust, including the transcripts from the Nuremberg trials as well as the book on which this film is based. The film would not tell me anything new; rather, it would most likely have the effect of leaving me upset and somewhat numb for several days. I do not need to put myself through this, regardless of the artistic merits of the film. I am already very sensitized to human suffering and depravity, regularly coming into contact with the victims of all kinds of abuse (albeit at less intense levels) and having immersed myself in trying to understand the roots and causes of the horrific cruelty exhibited during the Third Reich. More recently on a visit to Prague I was invited by a friend to accompany him to Auschwitz concentration camp. Again I resisted because I knew I would be devastated emotionally for days. These are simple examples of the choice to protect myself from being hurt by an experience that was unnecessary in terms of my development, either intellectually or emotionally. For others, the film might have a different and perhaps positive effect giving a person perspective on some aspects of human nature, or maybe for others heightening a political vigilance because of the increased likelihood that a similar type of genocide could occur in this generation. Or then again, some may find benefit by becoming more aware of the place moral choice takes in the wider scheme of the human story. The central issue here is the meaning that an event has for us. We should not choose to suffer if we can see no meaning or benefit in it. If we use this as a benchmark when confronted with choice, we can significantly reduce the level of painful events in our lives, often leaving us braver and stronger when we have to deal with suffering that is necessary, unavoidable and/or meaningful. It also means that when we seek to enjoy ourselves, we are not as burdened with the worries and concerns that so often intrude and spoil opportunities for being free and playful.

Developing a Sense of Humour

The ability to laugh is a defining characteristic of human beings. It is self-transcendent, because it utilises the human ability to see ourselves in situations rather than be fully immersed in them. Once we have the experience of laughing about something, we have already scored a victory over it. This does not mean that we should trivialise what is important, but rather that where possible we can learn to see the funny and sometimes absurd aspects of how we operate in the world. Usually when we are in the midst of a crisis nothing seems funny about it, yet as it resolves and with some distance in time we can focus on some humorous incidents that made up the crisis. It is the ability to select these aspects that helps us to get beyond the immediate impact of painful experiences. A sense of humour can he developed by finding things to smile about. If we behave childishly in a situation, we can learn to smile at our antics rather than always focus on whether we were right or wrong, or in assigning blame to ourselves and others. Much of what human beings do when in trouble can be seen as rather ludicrous with the benefit of hindsight.

Recreation

Recreation is the adult word for play. It refers to creating and partaking in activities that help the individual to forget their woes, to experience freedom from the rough-and-tumble of everyday life and to give the body and mind a chance to heal. Unfortunately, many people cannot play without turning the event into competition, where their fragile egos are under threat if they feel that they could lose the game. In that case, it is better to play at activities that are not competitive, such as learning some new recreational skill, passive entertainment such as film or theatre (staying away from disturbing events, at least for a time). Enjoying the company of others by sharing activities such as concerts, hill-walking, dancing and a whole host of other possibilities depending on the individual's taste and time of life. When recreation is a regular part of one's life, then there are more resources to deal with the ongoing challenges and sometimes painful emotional experiences that are an in-built part of recovery.

This may all seem mere common sense and, of course, it is. But damaged people often find it difficult to establish a balance in their everyday lives. They have a tendency to complicate the simple things and sometimes to underestimate the intricacies of more complex elements in life. Learning how to play provides people with the distance needed to evaluate in a fresher frame of mind many of the issues that surround their lives. One of these issues is the enormously important area of learning new ways to build and sustain healthy relationships.

Building Healthy Relationships

One of the greatest challenges in healing a damaged childhood is building a new relationship to love. This is because one of the first and major distortions that occurs in a dysfunctional home is a destruction of the child's understanding and experience of love. A damaged person often does not know how to give and receive love in a healthy and wholesome way. In general, the distortion of love is expressed in one of three ways: an over-investment in love for others at the expense of a healthy love for oneself; a deep-seated dependence and neediness for continual affirmation from others; and an inability to experience any form of intimacy.

Usually, the kind of 'love' relationship a damaged person who is not in recovery chooses will be based on his or her typical way of coping with life. These relationships will largely be based on the destructive and life constricting patterns that have ensured the person's survival, but which offer little or no potential for real change and growth. Thus, the individual who 'copes' with life through active addiction tends to have friends and a partner who enable his addiction by covering up, tolerating unacceptable behaviour, or even joining in the escapism of addiction with him. Those whose survival strategies include a high tolerance for suffering, as well as a need to 'fix' others, will tend to choose relationships with people who use them and who are themselves wounded.

Others who use dominance and achievement as primary coping strategies will tend to choose relationships with those who will not challenge them, and who tend to be passive and dependent. Often the dynamics of these types of relationships are confused with love, but it is distorted love, which leads to further constriction and lack of development. For damaged people, the realm of love is a minefield. More specifically, the adage that 'opposites attract' is often a recipe for disaster. In some situations, the attraction to the opposite qualities in another is evidence that the core distorted emotions and the survival strategies are in place and that the other person is being used, often unconsciously, to compensate for the weakness and defects in a person's own development. Furthermore, in such situations these deficiencies will remain unchallenged and perhaps become even more exacerbated in the relationship. In recovery, a different basis for love is needed. This is true whether it be romantic love or platonic friendship.

I recently had a therapeutic conversation with a client that brought much of this into bold relief. This woman, in her middle forties, had spent twenty-five years in an unhappy marriage and was still trying to find a way to change her partner so that she could live with him in some degree of peace. I asked her how she went about buying a pair of shoes. After looking rather surprised at the question, she described herself trying on a new pair, testing them for size, looking at the colour and deciding if they match the outfit for which they were intended, and finally looking at how much they cost and if she could afford them. Then I asked her to apply this simple process of decision making to her current relationship. A look of dawning insight, combined with sadness, crossed her face as she saw that she had never really evaluated her relationship in terms of what it was doing to her; nor had she perceived that her rights and needs are very important issues that need to be taken into account in her choice of who to live with. It is amazing how many damaged people give the purchase of a pair of shoes, which cost a less than a hundred euros and can be discarded easily, more careful examination than the relationship in which they will invest enormous emotional energy and to which they will devote a huge part of their lives.

In the process of recovery, it is often essential for the individual to examine the kinds of relationships in which he or she invests. Healthy relationships are those that offer the individual a loving context, in which he or she is challenged to continue to explore and develop his or her personality, while enjoying the friendship and companionship of another along the way. Some of the key issues in such relationships are: desire, trust, mutuality, challenge and compatibility.

Desire

Desire is one of the key emotional elements in a healthy relationship. It is usually thought of in terms of sexual attraction, but it is in fact a much more global phenomenon. A deep non-sexual relationship is marked out by the individual's desire for the companionship of the other. This desire is felt as a wanting to be close in companionship, to share thoughts and feelings with the other, and to want to get to know his or her thoughts and feelings. The relationship becomes sexual when the partners wish to share each other's bodies to give and receive sexual pleasure and the intense closeness that such an encounter can provide. In all such relationships, there are times when desire fades for a time. When this happens, many damaged people become afraid, for it is a common experience for people in recovery to find it difficult to leave relationships. When desire fades, the possibility of the relationship ending comes into view, causing anxiety to those in the relationship. This is particularly acute when it happens to only one of the individuals. It is important to recognise that emotional fluctuations are a normal part of any relationship. If, however, the feeling of wanting to be with someone changes and lasts for a long period, then the relationship is in trouble. Whether the relationship can recover depends to a large extent on the other factors listed above. The first of these is trust.

Trust

Trust is perhaps the toughest and most challenging aspect of any relationship. Damaged people have enormous difficulty with trust. This difficulty takes two forms. The first is a naive trust in others, regardless of whether or not they deserve it. This happens to people when their sense of their own needs and rights are continually made subservient to those of others. Often starved emotionally, the trusting individual accepts any crumb of love and affection given by another. This leads to the scenario whereby the individual is easily manipulated by anyone who wants to use them. Rather than face up to the pain involved in recognising the lack of real love by those with whom they are involved, they deny it by making excuses and minimising the effects of the relationship on her well-being. This denial is often underpinned by a fear of loss. Such a fear is often an echo of all the unresolved losses that the individual has yet to resolve and let go. I have dealt in detail with this subject in Chapter 7. Until a person has dealt with her losses, they will continually intrude upon and interrupt her ability to find a healthy trust in a relationship.

The second difficulty with trust is that of an inability to trust anyone - including oneself - at a deep level. This is a more common experience, which damaged people confront as they try to build healthy relationships with others. Having learned early in life to put their armour on and to protect themselves from the hurts inflicted in destructive families, or in ill-treatment at school, they carry this vigilant untrusting attitude into their adult relationships. Many will as a result flit from one relationship to another, and run away the moment they feel themselves becoming exposed. Others will hide in a safe relationship, where they know that the other person does not have the keys necessary to unlock their secret selves. In both circumstances, there is a great deal of emotional dissatisfaction and a chronic sense of emptiness. One of the important elements in overcoming this problem is honesty. The armour a damaged person uses consists of secrecy, pretence, lying through fear and running away. Honesty dismantles these protective layers. It is a paradox that one can learn trust by being honest.

Most people think that you have to trust someone before you can be honest with them. This, in my experience, is erroneous where damaged people are concerned. A damaged person who has difficulty trusting is not going to trust without learning to take a risk. Nobody has learned to swim without getting into the water; similarly, no one has learned to trust without first putting themselves on the line. And like swimming, one can gradually test the water, until one feels safe enough to go in the deep end. In a relationship, a person can take small risks with honesty, gradually making larger strides in the journey of becoming transparent to those with whom he or she cultivates friendship.

It is important to clarify here that I am speaking of close personal friendship, and ultimately the cultivation of abiding love - whether or not this has a sexual component. In these areas, it is also important to note that when damaged people take a risk with honesty, they may need to run away for a period until they have time to sense gradually that the recipient of their trust is not going to hurt or reject them. Obviously, every time a damaged person risks honesty and is met with rejection, they will have more difficulty next time, which is how the difficulty with trust developed in the first place. However, there is no other road, and in recovery one can learn to discover those people with whom this rejection is less likely to happen. One of the characteristics to look out for in this regard is mutuality.

Mutuality

Mutuality refers to the balance of give and take in a relationship. We have seen earlier that damaged people place themselves in relationships that are not mutual. Either the individual gives consistently with little attention to his own needs, or he is dependent and relies too heavily on the other, failing to take sufficient responsibility for himself. A healthy relationship, on the other hand, is one in which both people invest in each other, give and receive from each other. How this operates will change from time to time, especially if one person becomes particularly needy or vulnerable for a time. In this case, the other person may take a lead role in being strong or capable, until such time as the vulnerable one has found a way through his or her particular dilemma.

An important issue in regard to mutuality in a relationship is the notion of unconditional love. For some people - the more idealistic among us - unconditional love is a notion that one person can love another without condition for the lifetime of a relationship. This is to my mind erroneous when it comes to the kind of relationships that I am discussing here. A personal relationship between two people is based on the foundation that each is enriched, develops and grows as a direct result of being involved with the other. Without the effort and contribution of both people, the relationship will stagnate and die.

Certain types of relationships require unconditionality. The relationship between a parent and a young child is a good case in point. It is this unconditional quality that provides the child with a foundation on which to develop trust that continues on into adulthood. Another example of unconditionality is that which characterises charitable relationships, where people give of themselves out of their own bounty, without expecting anything in return. But these relationships are not friendships and, while they have an important role in the human story, they are not the basis for friendship or lover relationships. We should not confuse love with pity or charity in the special close relationships that most human beings need in order to be fulfilled or happy. Our expectations in relationships are important, and need to be acknowledged.

In some instances where damaged people are concerned, however, these expectations can be unrealistic and could not be met by any relationship. This occurs particularly when that person is trying, within the context of an adult relationship, to compensate for losses that occurred early in life. A good example of this occurs when an adult wants to have a relation ship that will make up for his or her loss of a healthy love relationship with either parent. Stereotypical examples of this abound in opposite sex relationships, where the man wishes to turn his partner into his mother, or the woman wishes her partner to provide a fatherly relationship. No adult relation ship can do this without ultimately becoming destructive to both people. This is so because the person will have idealised what a mother or father figure can be and because, to a large extent, the partner who tries to fit these roles will have to be perfectly unconditional in their love for the one demanding from them. The roots of this type of difficulty deserve some clarification.

Children are by nature thoroughly needy, narcissistic and self-centred, especially during the early years of childhood. If they do not have these needs met and are expected or forced to surrender them too soon, then the adults who emerge will carry many narcissistic needs for unconditional love into their adult relationships. When this happens, several characteristics emerge in the ebb and flow of close personal contact with others. Outbursts of rage (an adult version of a temper tantrum), extreme possessiveness, jealousy, sulking and continual need for attention are all evidence of the child's narcissistic needs exploding into the adult relationship.

Damaged people usually have to confront these problems in learning how to build healthy, mutually fulfilling relationships with others. A central element in navigating these emotional storms is that of recognising one's responsibility to learn how to grow up and live with unmet needs, rather than focusing on the deficiencies of a partner unable to meet these needs in a consistent and unconditional manner. This brings us to another important aspect of a healthy relationship: Challenge.

Challenge

A healthy adult relationship is one which challenges both parties to come to terms with their weaknesses and find mature ways to grow beyond them. An unhealthy relationship can often be marked out by a willingness of one person to tolerate too much, and the other to fail to accept deficiencies and weaknesses in himself. In this scenario, the tolerant person fails to challenge the partner, and ends up swallowing his frustration and anger. The other person ends up denying his faults, often projecting blame for his weakness onto his friend or partner. This type of unhealthy relationship is in essence a collusion between two people to maintain the status quo, and does not provide the opportunity for growth and change within the context of that relationship.

An important element in whether or not a relationship provides a challenge to the individuals in it is the degree to which both people have a firm sense of their own identity. When this is the case, both of them have a reasonably clear sense of their direction in life, ambitions, values and desires. Neither is looking to the other for an answer to these developmental issues and both, as a result, can provide an ongoing sense of growth and change as each person seeks to continue in what Carl Jung calls the process of individuation - that is, becoming an individual and exploring life from that standpoint. True intimacy comes about when two people share in this process, and provide love, support and respect for each other as they continue to grow in their own sense of individuality. When there is failure to accept the challenges to grow and mature by both people, there is a tendency to spend their energies trying to make each other change into someone they are not, and perhaps could never be. It is in this arena that the issue of compatibility becomes crucial for the long-term survival of the relationship.

Compatibility

Contrary to the notion that opposites attract and that good relationships are in general found with people who are very different in major elements of personality and beliefs, it is more likely that sustaining, healthy relationships are found among those who have a great deal in common, with just enough diversity to keep the relationship interesting. If we accept that a healthy relationship is based on two people having a clear sense of their own identities, sharing with each other on the journey through life, it becomes clear that the people must have a lot in common. It is this common ground in a relationship that is called compatibility. The following areas are of particular relevance where compatibility is concerned: intellectual equality; similarity in values; emotional harmony; and, with regard to a lover relationship, sexual accord. Most good relationships reflect compatibility in each of these areas; some can sustain a major difference in one of these, but very few will survive a major difference in more than one.

Before briefly discussing each of these, it is necessary to remind the reader that I am speaking of people who are reasonably intact within themselves. Compatibility alone does not mean that a relationship is a healthy one. A very sick relationship can be a very compatible one. Take, for example, a relationship between two people who rely totally on intellectual or religious pursuits to the exclusion of the other dimensions of relationship. These could be said to be very compatible, but neither person grows in the other important elements of human development within the context of the relationship. Furthermore, when one of the pair begins to make radical changes as a result of a personal crisis, the other will either try to suppress this development, retreat from the relationship, or in some cases recognise that they too need to work on themselves. In this latter situation, the relationship may become healthier and be sustained. In the former instances, the relationship may continue in its constricted form as a result of the abdication of one of the partners, or the relationship will end.

Intellectual Equality

One of the most popular notions surrounding what makes a good, healthy relationship is that of communication. And of course, this is true. What is not so apparent is that good communication requires similar levels of intellectual functioning. People can have radically different ideas, and yet have very stimulating and interesting conversations. It is well-nigh impossible, however, for two people to have such stimulating experiences within a relationship if one is analytical and quick in his or her thinking and the other uninterested and avoids developing a thoughtful approach to life. There is, of course, a very wide range of possibilities when it comes to the level of intellectual focus that people bring to experience. Some are very content with a bare minimum of analytical thought, whilst other examine everything under an intellectual microscope. Where any one person finds him or herself along this range does not militate against a satisfactory relationship. What is essential is that the partners in a relationship share some similarity in their level of intellectual functioning. Without that, they will have little common ground on which to communicate.

Similarity in Values

A person's values comprise what he or she upholds as important in life, and also his or her moral beliefs concerning right and wrong. These beliefs (not just intellectual ideas, but also emotionally potent concerns) are like the tracks of a railway line. They guide a person's journey through life in much the same way that the tracks guide a train to its destination. When people share many common values, then their life journey is parallel and going in roughly the same direction. When peoples' values differ considerably, they may find themselves travelling in different directions and sometimes taking an opposite course. For a long-term relationship to be sustained, a great deal of common ground with regard to the values of the individuals in the relationship is needed.

Some examples may help to clarify this. The most common values concern the role of money and financial security, the importance of social status, religious beliefs, the importance of work, the level of order in the environment and the functioning of family. Major differences between people in relation to any of these areas usually lead to conflict. Sometimes compromises can be reached, but the greater the level of divergence, the less likely it will be that the relationship can continue without high levels of tension and stress. This is particularly so in relationships where people choose to live together and share in creating a family. It can be said that when it comes to wide divergence of values, the old adage that love conquers all is no longer valid.

Emotional Harmony

This is perhaps the most crucial area of compatibility. Emotional harmony refers to the way the people in a relationship deal with feelings. It is also the area where people can listen to and learn a great deal from each other - that is if they choose to. Each person comes into a relationship with a unique set of experiences and a set of needs, expectations and rules (often unconscious) as to how a relationship works in terms of fulfilling these needs. Emotional harmony means that there is some accord between the people in this regard. Some individuals, for example, need and want to give and receive a lot of affection. It is difficult for such a person to feel satisfied in a relationship with someone who finds affection difficult. In this situation, the person who is frightened of or uncomfortable with affection can find a great deal of joy in learning its value.

In other situations, one individual may like to talk a lot about feelings, whereas the partner may be inclined to keep feelings locked away. Again, there is much to be gained from learning to become more comfortable in speaking about feelings. If such changes do not occur, each partner can be left feeling alone, rejected and uncomfortable. The affectionate person feels emotionally starved, whilst his or her partner may feel pressured and uncomfortable, becoming even more withdrawn. Similarly, the talkative person can feel isolated and taken for granted if the partner does not at least listen encouragingly.

When people find themselves in relationships where the emotional elements are at odds with each other, they may need to address this problem with the help of counselling. It should be said, however, that counselling does not have any magic potions, and in some situations emotional incompatibility may be impossible to redress. In such a situation, the people in the relationship may choose to live with the unmet needs and focus on other aspects of the relationship that are fruitful and satisfying. In other circumstances, the relationship becomes painful and intolerable and will gradually erode until it is, to all intents and purposes, dead. It is an important element in building healthy relationships to understand the basic emotional needs of the individual. This is particularly so in choosing a partner, because ultimately most relationships can survive and grow when this part of a relationship works reasonably well.

Sexual Accord

It is worthwhile to point out that sexual difficulties are in most cases a result of a malfunction in some other aspect of the relationship. If, for example, a person feels taken for granted, lonely and inferior to his or her partner, it is very difficult for that individual to respond freely in the sexual aspect of the relationship. Sexual difficulties can also be encountered as a direct result of the sexual formation of one of the individuals, say for example as a result of sexual abuse, or over-moralistic and rigid teaching about the human body (a problem endemic to our culture until recently).

Having said that, however, there is also a place for discussing sexuality for its own sake. Sexual accord refers to some level of agreement (often unspoken) between partners as to the role and function of sex in the relationship. More specifically, there are two aspects to sexual activity where sexual harmony can founder. The first relates to the reality that sexual needs are a basic part of healthy living, and are not always connected and related to love and intimacy. They exist as part of the biological make up of human beings. The second element is that sexual needs are also connected to a couple's deep emotional interchange and communication. When there is a great divergence between the expression of these two aspects of sexuality in a relationship, then sexual harmony begins to founder. Take, for example, the common occurrence where one partner can only feel comfortable in sexual activity when it is surrounded with love and romance, whilst the other experiences it as primarily a release of physical sexual tension. In this situation, the former can feel used as a sex object, whilst the other may feel that it is shameful just to want sex without having all the emotional aspects present. When this problem is a constant feature of a sexual relationship, the issue needs to be addressed, because both partners have an unbalanced and unhealthy attitude to sexuality.

In a healthy relationship, there is a realisation that both elements of sexual expression have a part to play. Some sexual encounters are mainly a giving and receiving of physical pleasure, whilst others are deeply intimate and emotional. The balance between these two forms of expression is accepted as part of the relationship. Sexual harmony means that the individuals in the relationship have found ways to accommodate their differing needs at different times.

Thus far, this chapter has examined three crucial areas where changing actual behaviours are important in the process of recovery and growth. Getting help often is a very important step. Learning to enjoy and celebrate the fun elements of life, as well as pursuing healthy relationships, are equally import ant. There remains one significant area in most peoples' lives that also requires evaluation, and sometimes change, in order for them to carve out a fulfilling and rich experience of life: work and career.

Re-evaluating One's Career

One of the central planks of most people's lives is their work. This includes those whose main career is that of building a home and the care of children. Furthermore, as we have seen in the early part of this book, early influences have long-term effects on every aspect of one's life, including the paths we take in relation to work. Recovery and growth, therefore, often involve taking a close look at the reasons why one has chosen a particular career path.

It is a common occurrence that people who have experienced neglect, hurt and trauma in their family of origin or in their experiences of school have been profoundly affected in the way that their career development has proceeded. I have spoken earlier of the problems of loss of self-esteem and confidence that afflict many who have endured such experiences. The consequences of this are often an important part of where they find themselves as adults. Many people who lost confidence at a young age were unable to concentrate or achieve within the educational system, and as a direct result found their prospects for work extremely limited. They may be bright and competent people, who find themselves in dead-end jobs, or unemployed. Others, who used popularity and academic achievement as the only basis for self-worth, can find themselves in highly stressful work that provides social status and financial rewards, but causes untold hard ship to their emotional and spiritual well-being, as well as indirectly affecting their families.

As I write this, I am keenly aware that economic circumstances in society determine to a large extent the accessibility for change in relation to work. That being said, however, there is much to be gained by examining the nature of one's work and in seeking to consider its relevance and suitability. Many people find that the reasons why they were attracted to a particular line of work may no longer be relevant, and that large areas of their personality and abilities are not being utilised. A useful way of understanding how this comes to pass is in examining the particular roles that individuals take in their family of origin, and how they tend to reflect these roles in the way their working lives develop. Let us look at a few examples (the family roles presented in these examples are discussed in detail in my earlier book, Alcoholism and the Family).

Paula was the 'lost child' in her family of origin. She is a successful administrator in a state-run organisation. She is well paid and has risen gradually through a series of promotions. She is very responsible and effective in her work. The problem is that she hates her job. When we examined what attracted her to the work in the first place, several themes emerged. As the daughter of an alcoholic father, she wanted to get out of school as soon as possible and away from his influence. While she did well enough in her final school exams to earn a scholarship, she decided against further education, as it would keep her dependent to some degree on her father. She also wanted to be able to relieve the family from financial hardship by becoming independent. Another influence for her was the desire for financial security, even if it meant compromising about the kind of work she would really like to do. This need for financial security was grounded in her experience of fear, poverty and hardship that resulted directly from her father's alcoholism. Thus, someone with the intelligence, interest, desire and the academic background suited to follow a profession that she would have succeeded in, made a choice against her long-term fulfilment for reasons that should have had no part to play in her career path. Now, sixteen years later and after substantial recovery work, she is studying and training to be a psychologist.

Jennifer was a family caretaker. She took responsibility for all the misery and pain that went on in her family of origin. Like many such people, it is only a short step to seek out work in a caring profession (where else can you get paid for continuing what was a dysfunctional role in an otherwise very worthy career?). So she trained to be a nurse and married an alcoholic (an amazingly common phenomenon). Gradually, her life came apart and she had to stop working. In the space of a few years, Jennifer lost whatever tenuous confidence she had, until she herself fell prey to alcoholism. In recovery, she had to rebuild her career slowly and painstakingly, embarked on a university course, and is gradually setting out on a new career path.

John left school early because of family hardship. The oldest son in a large family, he left behind his schooling, where he was highly successful. After working in a factory for ten years and as the responsibility to his family became less taxing, he went back to school part time, got his final exams and continued on the path he should not have had to leave. He is now a successful professional with a doctorate degree.

Patrick was another family hero. He loved to achieve and be the centre of attention. Competing fiercely in all his exams, he came through schooling with flying colours. It was a natural step for him to seek out a profession where he could have financial success and more admiration from others. He chose a career in law, a highly prestigious job with financial rewards. Driving himself harder and harder from one success to another, trying to allay a deep feeling of insecurity and low self-esteem, all his attempts to quell his inner angst failed, as he found his success hollow and his life suffused with loneliness. All his artistic talent lay dormant and uncultivated, until he began to evaluate how his life was really turning out. Gradually he began to look at reducing his workload and to explore creative writing and landscape painting. In finding a more peaceful way of life, Patrick also discovered love and true companionship. He is not as successful a lawyer today, but he is a far more successful human being.

Peter was the family jester. He created fun for those around with all his acting out and irresponsibility. He had charm and wit, but no sense of his responsibility to himself. Lacking in concentration, paying scant attention to the need for endurance, he finished schooling with the bare minimum in his final examinations. This did not prevent him from becoming a successful salesman. His ready wit and charm served him well. His work also allowed him access to large amounts of cash, which was too big a temptation, given his proclivity to bet on horses. After embezzling a great deal of money, he found himself facing a prison sentence. This had the effect of focusing his attention on his irresponsibility and escapism. After much difficult recovery work, Peter has confronted his compulsive need for excitement and distraction and begun to find a greater inner peace, reflected in being able to work at tasks that require concentration and endurance.

These examples show how people can be cast into circumstances around the issue of work that are not really suitable for their needs. They also show that, with time, energy and commitment, people can and do change the direction of their working lives. This is something that many people find hard to believe and accept. They feel trapped by their career; to some extent this can be because of their financial commitments. Change, therefore, can take a lot of time and effort. But most importantly, one must believe that such change is possible. This is the first step in making such changes.

The second step involves getting a better understanding of the direction that a career change should take. There is little point in contemplating such change unless some clear sense of direction takes place. There are services available that help people to identify the kinds of work best suited to them. These usually focus on the three areas of career that need to be examined in finding some new direction: one's abilities, skills and personality. Professional help will enable a person to relate these areas to a particular career path, and show what areas of retraining and education are involved.

Naturally, there may need to be a degree of compromise as to how change can come about. In many situations, a person may need to accept some retraining for work that approximates their basic career orientation. Imagine, for example, someone who would like to become a social worker, but cannot organise - for whatever reason - the training necessary. He or she may have to settle for some kind of voluntary work, or work that allows caring contact with people without the need for a professional qualification. Change, therefore, may mean compromise. One of the benefits available in present-day society is the possibility for ongoing education for adults. The variety of training courses, both full time and part time, make it a real possibility for people to begin to explore learning new skills, even while continuing in their present work. I have seen this advance in society provide real opportunities for people whose career path was seriously undermined by emotional damage in early life.

We do not live in an ideal world, and this means that opportunities can be difficult for those who realise that their chosen work direction is unsuitable for them. It is, however, an important part of recovery and growth to examine this area. Most people spend a great deal of their productive energy at work. Whether one organises voluntary activity or seeks to retrain, the new direction takes a person out of the trap that he has found himself in as a legacy of his developmental history.

Caring for One's Body

The final section on doing things differently is learning how to care for one's body. Many damaged people allow their health to deteriorate. They do so by feeding their body with junk and unhealthy food, by not eating regularly, by giving it toxic substances, by not remaining fit and not having enough rest. All of this can be further exacerbated by the presence of unhealed emotional conflicts and stress. Many of the areas of healing discussed above will have a direct impact on the care of the body. Less stress and internal pain, renewed hope and confidence and many other areas of change generally bring about a more positive and nurturing attitude to one's life. When these changes are in place, it becomes a lot easier to tackle many of the bodily symptoms of emotional damage - addiction, overweight, restlessness and so on. Making a commitment to small changes in one's health becomes easier. Without these changes, many resolutions for change will fail, leading to frustration and hopelessness.

I am sceptical of the value of health fads and the resolutions people make in response to them. Dieting is a good case in point. Most people who go on diets end up putting back on the weight that they often so torturously lost, and in the process have usually done some damage to their body. The underlying emotional and psychological reasons for their ill health need to be addressed, before such changes can have a hope of being sustained. There is an enormous amount of information and guidance available in relation to physical health, and it is unnecessary to repeat the specifics here.

Summary

This chapter has focused on the primary areas where changes in what we do need to occur. It has looked at the issue of getting help in some detail, because it is often a crucial part of getting the clarity and direction needed to make best use of the process of recovery and growth. Having fun and learning to play are also an important part of being a healthy and fulfilled person. Building healthy relationships helps in healing many of the scars left by relationships that were damaging and destructive. Such relationships also promote continued development. Evaluating the nature of one's work and its effects on the quality of life are also areas to be addressed in recovery.

Whilst change may be difficult, it is possible to compromise and seek out some changes toward a direction more suited to an individual's personality and abilities. And finally, my rather brief comments on caring for the body do not in any way minimise the importance of doing this. All of these changes can be integrated into the emotional healing and redirected thinking discussed in the earlier chapters. The final crucial area of recovery is also relevant to assist these changes. This is the area of spiritual growth.

CHAPTER 10
Spiritual Growth

*"The tragedy of life is not death but what we let die inside of
us while we live."*

Anthony de Mello

Introduction

Beginning this chapter challenges me in a similar fashion to the
beginning of the book. For a psychologist to speak about spiritual
matters is always a highly risky undertaking. This is because there are
others whose life's work centres on this subject and who can do it
greater justice. As a consequence, I am aware of my shortcomings in
discussing spiritual matters. A second reason for experiencing some
apprehension while setting out on this chapter lies in the standing
that spirituality holds in the minds of many psychologists, as well
as those heavily influenced by modern psychological thinking. For
scientific psychology and the more rationalistically minded, the
matters of the spirit are at best comforting illusions and at worst
an abject denial of reality. As a result, I will present here a brief
explanation for the inclusion of this chapter, as part of the position
that spirituality is of central importance to healing and recovery.

I am as sceptical and rationalistic as any of my colleagues. I have
a strong resistance to the notion of any forces exercising an influence
on human and natural life, other than those which can be measured
and explained scientifically. I think this resistance is very useful, for it
prevents me falling off the cliff into intellectual suicide and accepting
the validity of any experience based simply on a person's (including
my own) subjective interpretation. The lack of critical insight when
dealing with matters of the spirit leads to all kinds of quackery. My
scepticism, however, is a bias grounded in my education, and perhaps
a reflection of my own pride. Many people in the helping professions

have over the past few decades grown into an educated elite, who for some strange reason believe that the western world's concept of learning and knowledge is greater and more valid as a way of finding truth than any other approach. The great mistake in this is the failure to accept that the scientific method is only applicable to certain subject matters, namely the physical world. We have become experts in its use, and as a result are building a technological world as well as dismantling much of orthodox religion.

These two movements have brought very useful benefits, such as a better quality of life for many, the control of disease, and increased power of communication on one hand; and rejection of hypocrisy and elitism in the religious influences on peoples' lives on the other. The negative fall-out from these movements has yet, in my opinion, to be fully felt. The dehumanisation of people and the creation of an underclass whose social identity is lost is one I have mentioned earlier. These effects arise from an optimistic and naive belief in technological progress for its own sake.

A second series of effects lie in the loss of any spiritual understanding of the nature of human beings, and a lack of serious endeavour to provide people with resources and encouragement to care for and cultivate their spirituality. The diminished power of orthodox religion has left many people in a spiritual vacuum. This is in itself not a bad thing; because the alternative of a rationalistic, power structured hierarchy controlling the spiritual elements of development has caused untold damage to peoples' lives over the centuries, and is no longer acceptable to most thinking people. As yet, however, there is no clear replacement that provides for the spiritual hunger and the need for meaning in peoples' lives. The secular replacements of communism and fascism in the twentieth century make the Spanish inquisition look mild in contrast.

The remainder of this chapter is an effort to present some positive guidelines by which people can cultivate their spirituality and set out on a journey of spiritual growth and fulfilment. Several key themes emerge from my own experience and from observing those who have taken on the challenge of spiritual growth. Before examining these, it may be useful to clarify what spirituality is not.

What Spiritual Growth is Not

Spiritual growth is not a fine-tuning of an intellectual set of beliefs about the nature of the universe, the existence of God, or the truth claims of a particular religious orthodoxy. Such beliefs are often crucial in providing a context for a person's spiritual development, but in themselves are merely a cognitive frame through which the world is viewed. This is not to deny their importance. The idea of truth is important in evaluating any spiritual experience; and I am of the old school, which suggests that a rational foundation for one's experience is healthy and important. An example may help to clarify this point. Recently, I listened to a comedian tell the story of intellectual development in matters philosophical. He began by commenting on the derision that many people have toward archaic and simplistic views of the nature of the universe. He took as his example the notion, once held, that the world was balanced on the back of a huge turtle. He then went on to describe the enormous technological and scientific development that led to the 'new physics' explanation (elucidated by Stephen Hawkins), that the universe exploded out of an infinitesimally small particle which had infinitely high density. His joke was that it was easier in some ways to accept the turtle explanation!

The implications of this story are far-reaching in terms of how we proceed spiritually. More specifically, certain questions arise. Is there any link between what are called spiritual experiences and the nature of reality? Is this link important in making the experience valid, or does the experience stand alone, in itself, for itself? If we take the turtle story a bit further, it might be said that those who accept the turtle explanation might focus their spiritual journey on a search for an understanding of the mind of the turtle. Others, more materialistically minded, might focus their concerns on the question of how energy becomes matter. We are left with the question: is it important whether the turtle exists, just as long as our search gives us experiences that help in our lives? Answering 'no' to this question is one of the central planks of many who involve themselves in the spiritual journey; it is an approach which, I believe, leads to spiritual impoverishment. This is because once we separate the spiritual as belonging to the realm of experience only, and the nature of reality as belonging to the world of logic, we have created an artificial and somewhat schizophrenic approach to human experience.

Some writers explain this as a split between left- and right brain functioning. I am inclined to agree. The left brain is primarily useful for logical thinking, examining cause-and effect relationships and other types of reasoning. The right brain is the casket in which the world of fantasy, imagination and creativity resides. Granted, it is underused in the modern world, but just as overuse of left-brain approaches have brought enormous problems in its train, so too will the overuse of right-brain approach to life, at the expense of logic and reasoning.

It can be said, therefore, that a new approach which tries to combine the truths gleaned from those who endeavour to understand human spirituality with those of a more empirical and scientific bent is required. I believe that such an approach is in its infancy, and finds its expression in the work of those who are working specifically in the realm of spiritual healing. What we do not need is a cynical rejection of all things spiritual among those who lead the field in the main stream areas of psychiatry and psychology. Nor do we need a naive and simplistic acceptance of a fairy-tale world based on woolly thinking and lack of critical evaluation. Carl Jung grappled with this dilemma throughout his life. He concluded that human consciousness is still in a development phase that makes it impossible yet to fully harmonise these two worlds. He writes that "Psychic reality exists in its original oneness and awaits man's advance to a level of consciousness where he no longer believes in the one part and denies the other, but recognises both as constituent elements of one psyche

What is Spirituality?

Fundamental to the notion of spirituality is the recognition that human beings have a potential to experience profoundly altered states of consciousness. Such states have been known to open doors into realities that are different from those of ordinary, everyday experiences. Such ordinary experience is mediated in a conscious waking state by the senses of sight, hearing, smell and touch. Spiritual, non-ordinary states are mediated by other faculties, about which little is known. Part of the ignorance surrounding the capacities inherent in human beings for such experience is due to the rejection of their validity by the rationalistic, scientific culture that has dominated western thinking since the period known as the Enlightenment. This rejection was expressed most forcefully against those cultures and societies where these experiences were an intrinsic part of their function. They were colonised and suppressed by the more technologically developed powers, who in most cases saw these rituals and experiences as primitive expressions of magic, to be destroyed in the name of progress.

A second element in spirituality is the worldwide phenomenon of a desire among people to seek out self-transcendent experience, where there is a sense of loss of ego and a blissful connection to some reality that is greater than the practical, everyday world. Many believe this experience to be a connection with a transcendent being that we call God.

A third element in spirituality is the phenomenon of continued existence after bodily death (for some, this includes the notion of existence before birth). This belief, whilst bringing comfort to many in the wake of the loss of a loved one, is also a way of coping with the reality of one's own death. These emotional benefits are, however, only a part of the reason why people throughout the ages have held fast to the belief in some kind of afterlife. The teachings of most religions include some conception of an afterlife, and the concept of the resurrection is a central plank in Christian and Islamic theology. These teachings, as well as the many experiences of paranormal and ghostly occurrences, have added weight to the idea that human consciousness does not finish with the death of the body.

A fourth element of spirituality is the acceptance that forces both within human consciousness as well as outside this realm are at work in influencing certain events. These influences, when operated on the human experience, are called miracles. Obvious examples of such events abound, including the healing of the body against all the predictions of medical science. Others include experiences such as answered prayer and the protection of believing individuals in dire circumstances.

All the above can be explained away by those who cannot accept, for whatever reason, the existence of an alternative realm working outside normal human consciousness. Religious explanations, whilst acknowledging the reality of the above elements, differ greatly in the meanings they attach to them. It is not within the range of this book to examine these issues further, with the exception of saying that, in my opinion, some rules apply to the accuracy or inaccuracy surrounding what people believe. It is not enough simply to state that any old explanation will do. If a person believes in the existence of God, he or she has every right to do so; if on the other hand another person does not, he or she also has that right. It can be said, however, that they both cannot be correct in their view.

Similarly, people who believed that the world was flat had a right to the belief; those who believe that the world was round are also entitled to the belief. We now realise, however, that the world is round, and that those who believed differently were incorrect - regardless of how much comfort they took from the belief. The rise of modern science into the age of space exploration has provided more information on which to judge the accuracy of many beliefs about the natural world. In my view, these developments do not help to measure the accuracy of many spiritual beliefs. A different kind of endeavour is required, one which is only beginning and which will, if given sufficient support, see large advances in terms of our understanding of the spiritual world. Presently, however, we must be content with the little we know and operate outward from that knowledge if we wish to explore our own spiritual growth. Two general areas appear to be of value in this regard: cultivating a sense of the sacred and pursuing self-transcendence.

Cultivating a Sense of the Sacred

Part of growing spiritually involves developing a keener sense of the sacred. This can be a difficult task in modern life, with its continual busyness and emphasis on external activities. Sacredness refers to a type of reverence for the spiritual, a surrender to its power and letting oneself into a place of focus and quiet concentration on its meaning. Certain objects, or practices, become sacred by means of the attachment of meaning to them. Objects such as statues and paintings, and rituals such as prayer and benediction, hymns, meditations, holy books and music are not in themselves sacred. They become sacred through the inherent human ability to project meaning onto such things through symbolism. They then represent the sacred in a way that is accessible through ordinary consciousness. Thus, a picture of the Madonna and child can represent to some people the mystery of the birth of Christ; to others it can represent motherhood in all its depths; whilst still others see it in terms of a nurturing of the universe for the human being, as child. The picture itself, therefore, is not what is important. Its sacredness lies in the meanings projected onto it. It is this ability to symbolise sacredness that can be utilised in helping spiritual growth. Three areas of life seem to be particularly accessible to a sense of the sacred: 1. one's own existence; 2. the mystery of life itself; and 3. the mystery of the supernatural.

One's own Existence

In a world characterised on the one hand by technological advancement, the reduction of people to cogs in a fast-moving, profit oriented culture, materially cared for from cradle to grave; and on the other hand by those impoverished and abandoned societies where people live out a desperate struggle for physical survival, it is difficult for individuals to connect with the experience of their own existence as a miracle. And yet this connection is a profoundly important part of spiritual growth. When I speak of an individual's existence, I am not referring to the ego struggle to assert ones' control over the immediate environment. I mean a deeper experience, one which concerns the incarnation of life in a unique fashion in every human being. I can do no better here than quote from Thomas Moore, who writes in The Care of the Soul: Care of the soul... goes beyond the secular mythology of the self and recovers a sense of the sacredness of each individual life. This sacred quality is not just value - all lives are important. It is the unfathomable mystery that is the very seed and heart of each individual. Shallow therapeutic manipulations aimed at restoring normality or tuning a life according to standards reduces - shrinks - that profound mystery to the pale dimensions of a social common denominator referred to as the adjusted personality.

The sacredness of one's existence can so easily be forgotten, a passing shadow in an otherwise busy life, evoked momentarily and perhaps haplessly now and then, by some experience of extraordinary beauty or intimacy. As I write this, I look across at my young daughter, Sarah, and am taken away by the depth of love I have for her. The music from the soundtrack of the film The Mission plays quietly, and I realise how easy it is for me to acknowledge the mystery and wonder of her young life. But I too am a miraculous event, despite all my failings, wounds and mistakes. There is comfort and hope in this realisation. Spiritual growth involves taking an active interest in cultivating that sense of being a miracle. It has nothing to do with being a perfect person; it is not a self-improvement exercise, and to try and turn it into such an endeavour is a tawdry compromise.

I am reluctant to advise on specific ways in which a person can approach this part of spiritual growth, lest it be interpreted as a simple matter with a winning formula. Every person differs in the way that his or her sacredness can be experienced and expressed. Certain activities can encourage such expression, however, by providing a context for its appearance into conscious experience. One of these is that of contemplative focusing. A useful way to begin this is to take a short period each day, find a quiet place, light a candle and focus on what it means to be a carrier of life. Let the candle light symbolise the light of your own life; sit quietly, letting the experience of life flow through you. Doing this exercise regularly will begin to open doors to your spiritual life. Once this begins to happen, then new interest in matters of the spirit takes hold.

The Mystery of Life Itself

It is not unusual for those who cultivate their spirituality to become concerned for the way living creatures are treated. Many choose no longer to eat meat; others fight for the welfare of animals, for humane farming and so on. At times, some of these practices are taken to an extreme, and at others they become distorted and destructive. Animal rights activists who send letter bombs to politicians are, of course, seriously disturbed. These extreme elements are off-putting and tend to hide the truth: that growing spiritually means beginning to appreciate more deeply the mystery of life in all its forms. The leaf that falls in autumn renews the earth and provides food to sustain the new growth of spring; the continuing mystery of death and rebirth going on all around us is often ignored. And yet each of us is a small link in that circle of life. By focusing on life in nature, we can begin to gain a sense of our place in the wider circle. This helps us to lose an overdeveloped sense of our own importance and places many of the trials and tribulations of our lives in a more serene context.

One of my favourite activities, particularly during times of adversity, is to sit quietly near the seashore, preferably at night, when visual distraction is minimal. The constant movement of the tide along with the vastness of the ocean cultivates in me a sense of the timeless and the eternal. The ocean represents for me the nurturing power of life. Its teeming richness, its changing nature from quiet ebbing and flowing to passionate turbulence, creates a picture of the life force that generates all of life, my own included. When I moved away from access to the sea I can sit out on the porch on a starry night, all wrapped up in a blanket when the frost comes, and get lost in awesome expanse of the firmament. When we integrate these kinds of experiences into our lives in a consistent fashion, we draw closer to a sense of connection to forces that are transcendent.

The Mystery of the Supernatural

No discussion on the topic of spirituality would be sufficient without focusing on the issue of the supernatural. For many people, the central plank of spirituality lies in a belief in God. And whilst there are as many conceptions of God as there are believers, certain basic differences in belief about God can be seen to exist. In terms of spiritual growth, some aspects of the way people view God can be a hindrance to development. The one we are most familiar with in my own culture is that of a personal and punitive God, whose love must be earned and whose wrath must be assuaged through penance and good works. This is a God who doesn't like sex or too much fun, but seems pleased with sentimental piety and lack of passion, a God who is fundamentally insecure, because he gets angry if people don't believe in him.

Thankfully, the last few decades has seen a gradual erosion of the power invested in this kind of distorted spirituality and, in the light of the harm to the emotional, intellectual and spiritual development of people that occurred as a direct result of being indoctrinated with such a belief, it is better that such notions be dismantled. The question arises, however, as to what can replace such a destructive view of God for those people who wish to retain a religious sense of the Divine as part of their spiritual growth. Recent trends suggest that an alternative picture of God is being imported from eastern thought. This is particularly obvious among those who can be characterised as 'New Age'. This is a rather loose collection of generally sensitive and searching people who have rejected most of the tenets of the religion of their childhood. They have sought new beliefs, generally imported and westernised from the major eastern religions of Hinduism and Zen Buddhism. These beliefs include much that is magical, fairy tale-like and tolerant of almost all ways of understanding God.

In essence, God is seen in the non-personal realm of some kind of spiritual, intelligent force that is present in all life and embraces both good and evil. This viewpoint is essentially pantheistic, and it is perhaps one of the oldest and most primitive notions of God in human history. What is some what surprising is that this view is seen by many as new and radical. In response to this belief, C. S. Lewis makes a salient clarification:

Pantheism certainly is congenial to the modern mind; but the fact that a shoe slips on easily does not prove that it is a new shoe - much less that it will keep your feet dry. Pantheism is congenial to our minds, not because it is the final stage in a slow process of enlightenment, but because it is almost as old as we are. It may even be the most primitive of all religions... So far from being the final religious refinement,

Pantheism is in fact the permanent natural bent of the human mind; the permanent ordinary level below which sometimes man sinks, under the influence of priest craft and superstition, but above which his own unaided efforts can never raise him for very long.

Whilst there is much to be said for abandoning the damaging aspects of orthodoxy, and for embracing an experience based on a tolerant spiritual belief system, there are some pitfalls in much of the new age spirituality. My own opinions on this matter are that the God that a person needs as part of spiritual life must at least reflect the highest characteristics of humanity. No person can understand the nature of God, for if that was the case then that person would be God. All we can hope for is that our experience and our understanding reveal some reflection of the nature of God. In this respect, God must he greater than humanity in all the core characteristics that set human beings apart from the rest of nature. These characteristics are, I believe, the capacity for love, the ability of creative intelligence and a distinct identity.

One cannot have a relationship with a vague celestial energy force without attributing personal characteristic to it. Once that is done, we have made that force or power into something distinct and personal - in other words, a God. Much of our own religious heritage can he used to facilitate this area of spiritual growth. Having discarded its damaging elements, there remains in the orthodox a rich seam of spiritual nurturing in the rituals of contemplative prayer, symbolism of religious celebration and peaceful serenity of many religious practices. Those, however, who have been badly hurt through the 'sins' of orthodox religion may not be able to take part in any such involvements, and it is important that they do not try too hard in this regard. Any God worthy of worship must he of a nature to understand the hurts of people as well as secure enough not to take the rejection of hurt people as a mark against them. It is useful in this context to remember that some of the most spiritual people on earth have no identifiable religion, and that some of the most religious people on earth are awful. Thus, for some, an outright rejection of all the orthodox religious elements of their lives may be a temporary, or even permanent, part of a journey through healing and recovery.

Self-Transcendence

During my twenties, one of the subjects that engaged my attention was the nature of transcendent experience and its place in the development and personal growth of people. I was particularly intrigued by what I saw as a dialectic between self-actualisation and self-transcendence. Now, decades later, I remain keenly interested in these two processes as part of the human story.

Much of the psychological literature on self-development places primary emphasis on self-actualisation the individual's growth and expression of self in the world. It focuses on issues such as expressing one's potential, loving oneself, having a firm sense of one's identity and high self-esteem. Self-transcendence has a different focus, and has been the foremost element of much religious teaching throughout history. Its meaning is reflected beautifully in the words of Jesus Christ, when he says 'He who tries to save his soul shall lose it, and he who loses his soul for my sake shall find it.' The emphasis in transcendence concerns self-sacrifice, giving to others in material and non-material ways, and getting beyond the concerns with self.

Thus far, the content of this book has largely focused on the self-actualising elements of recovery and growth. This is because it is an essential part of the recovery process. Furthermore - and this is an important issue in terms of what I say about self-transcendence - it is dangerous to a person's development to pursue the self-transcendent elements of life without first having a healthy sense of self. Much of what I have written on the topic of co-dependence finds its roots in attempts by people to build self-transcendent attitudes and behaviours into their way of life before they have any developed sense of their own identity, and before learning a sense of self-protection. This process is often as a direct result of guilt-producing religious teachings, given to children before they have developed the maturity and inner strength necessary to integrate such concepts healthily into their lives.

Self-transcendence plays a key role in the kind of person who emerges through the healing process. Paul Tournier makes this explicit, when he says:

It is clear that whatever school of psychology is followed, free and loving self-giving always appears as the final objective which the psychotherapeutic treatment aims at making the person capable of achieving. The first movement, however, must be creation. This is the meaning of psychotherapy: the creation of the person. The second movement will be de-creation. The first is enrichment and possession, the second is shedding and detachment.

Similarly, Tournier says*: 'One must have a place before one can give it up. One must receive before giving, exist before abandoning oneself. We receive a place only so as to eventually leave it, treasure only to cast it away, a personal existence only so as to offer it up'.*

Having set out these protective points, we can move on to the core issue of what it means to develop self-transcendence as part of growing into a mature adult. A useful beginning is to take an example from theology, where it speaks of the character of God as being both immanent and transcendent. Immanence refers to God's active presence in the life of His creation, and His transcendence speaks of His being beyond and above His creation. Transcendence, therefore, means being beyond. I am using the word 'being' in the sense of existence. Transcendence is about existing beyond the mundane and the practical. Human beings have a capacity for experiencing existence as being beyond any particular condition of their lives.

There appear to be two general categories of transcendental experience; one is where the person's ego is experienced as present, but where its narcissistic needs are not the driving force. This form of transcendence is generally concerned with the act of loving others, of going the second mile, of self forgetfulness in dealing with people. They are often somewhat uncomfortable, in so far as the call of one's selfishness remains unheeded. The athlete who endures the pain of hitting the wall on a marathon run must choose to accept the pain for the higher goal of completing the task. In this simple example, he transcends himself. The human characteristic of freedom provides the crucial element in this category of transcendental experience.

The second category of transcendence has the central theme of a loss of ego boundaries. If we imagine our ego being enveloped with something akin to a psychological skin that contains all the experiences of the ego, the transcendent experience occurs when this skin breaks and the ego becomes lost into the experience. Three very common human experiences are characterised by this phenomenon - falling in love, sexual intimacy and ecstasy (religious or otherwise). Other types of transcendental experiences are profoundly painful and very frightening. These include psychotic breakdown, drug-induced paranoia, and what some theologians describe as demonic possession. The positive and euphoric aspects of transcendental experience are very tempting; because they can be induced artificially through drugs, they are an important consideration in understanding why certain people become addicts. Perhaps one of the best examples of this phenomenon is portray in the character of Tony Soprano in the last season of the massively successful show. After murdering Christopher, he travels to Florida to commiserate with one of his friends. After a dalliance with her she takes him out to the desert and they take a psychedelic drug (Ayahuasca) together. Tony has an epiphany. What seems so striking in this episode is that it shows that this psychopathic murderer still has the capacity for transcendent consciousness that seems completely unrelated to either his moral or personal maturity.

Several writers have recognised the connection between the spiritual experience of transcendence and the problem of addiction. Christina Grof and more recently Gabo Mate, for example, believe that addiction is in the main a spiritual problem, whereby the addict is continually attempting to create a transcendental experience and finds living within the boundaries of practical reality more and more painful. Theologian Adrian Van Kaam provided what is perhaps the most succinct, yet sophisticated, description of this phenomenon. In his view, the addict:

from the potential objects of addiction available to him within his situation he will select one that, according to his experience, takes him most completely out of the daily world of mastery, projects and responsibility, and which redeems him most effectively from his painful experience of impotence and emasculation. On the other hand, this object must grant him the deepest and most consistent experience of wholeness and fulfilment as a mere present. Soon the addict develops a magic belief in the object of his addiction; it becomes a powerful symbol of salvation and redemption from this unbearable world of impotence and failure. This almost mystical symbolism bestows on the object of addiction its excessive strength and its stubborn resistance to counter influence.

I have much sympathy with this view of addiction, particularly in consideration of the phenomenon known among heroin addicts as 'chasing the dragon'. Once the addict has experienced the rush of the first heroin high, he is unable to live in the grey world of reality; he continually tries to recreate the experience, even if in reality he is suffering the most awful traumas in the attempt.

It does appear that the use of drugs opens up both the positive and euphoric elements of transcendence, as well as the traumatic and terrifying ones. Perhaps all addictions are to some extent a distortion of the need for transcendental experience in human beings, and there are many implications for recovery from addiction in this view. So, like all crucial areas of human life, transcendence is open to distortion and destruction. Co-dependency - which as we have seen is a form of addictive relationship - appears to be a distortion of the first area of transcendence, that of transcending oneself for the sake of another. Addiction to mood-altering substances can be seen as a distortion of the second element, that of creating ego-less and euphoric experiences.

Where, then, lies the healthy development of transcendence? I have suggested above that two areas of transcendence exist, one where the person is consciously self-aware of themselves and the other where there is a loss of ego boundaries and an experience of ego loss. In both of these areas it is possible to pursue a healthy transcendental aspect of spiritual growth.

Self-Transcendence in the Presence of the Ego

While there may be many ways in which transcendence can exist in the presence of the conscious ego, three elements appear to be of substantial importance to spiritual growth: practicing love; forgiveness; and making amends.

Practicing Love

Practicing love means consciously setting out to improve one's ability to care for the needs and growth of others. It may seem somewhat unusual to think of love as something that needs practice. This is because many people confuse sympathy, as well as romantic attraction, with love. Whilst these are valid parts of the story of human love, they are not a necessary part of its existence. Many recovering people need to learn a new relationship to love. I have examined this topic in the narrow field of friendships and lover relationships. Part of spiritual growth, however, includes the broader dimensions of love, namely love of one's neighbour and for life in general. These elements of love require practice.

A useful guide in this process is to focus on how to expand the generous and self-giving aspects of one's character. Some people find it useful to take a few moments in each day to consider the needs of others, be they friends, associates, or just other people of whom one is aware. Having chosen a particular person, or set of people, plan some kind of action that may be of use or service to their needs. This may simply be a time to pray for them, to think kindly of them, or to do some practical service such as a phone call with a word of encouragement, sending a card or gift, or providing in some material way. Clearly, some sensitivity is required in this matter, because the welfare of another is the central concern. By practicing this kind of care and generosity, a person begins to experience a freedom from self that is an important part of being healthy and fulfilled. It is an undeveloped theme in most therapy, because as we have seen, the focus of therapy is primarily on building a self.

Forgiveness

Forgiveness is a second strand of the transcendent element of spirituality. Many people carry with them a cup of bitterness locked away in their hearts. It is usually there as a result of hurts visited upon them by others, and which they have not yet resolved. In some cases, a person moves towards attempts at forgiveness before having completed the work of grieving discussed in Chapter 6. When this happens, it is likely that forgiveness is being used as a form of repression or denial, and the bitterness and anger go underground, often to emerge in other situations or in other relationships. It is essential therefore to preface this discussion on forgiveness by acknowledging the importance of fully experiencing the feelings of hurt and grief that surround resolving our wounds. When this work is done, the person will be inhibited in his or her spiritual growth if he or she cannot forgive those who have caused hurt; and it is usually the case that an inability to forgive is grounded in a lack of healing.

What, then, is forgiveness? Two elements that have been associated with forgiveness provide some useful guidelines: understanding and cleansing. The phrase 'to understand is to forgive' may not always be true, but it does carry some validity. When we understand that those who hurt us are often themselves hurt people, sometimes acting in ignorance, other times acting out of their own dysfunction, it helps to distance us somewhat from the effects of their abuse. It is possible to separate the person from the act, and to acknowledge that when someone wounds us he or she also has other, kinder and better traits. No person is fully contained in any particular act. This is, of course, cold comfort for those whose lives have been tragically damaged as a result of the abuse of others. And yet it is an important step on the road of forgiveness. Forgiveness in this discussion is not for the benefit of the other person; it is for self-growth and the freedom of no longer carrying bitterness and pain within.

Understanding also contains within it the reality that no individual is without flaws, and that the one who is wounded can also wound. I believe that the teachings of Christ have tremendous wisdom in helping us to understand the nature of forgiveness. I am reminded here of the story where the Pharisees came to test Christ by presenting a woman caught in the act of adultery and who, under the old law of Moses, would be deemed punishable by stoning. The wisdom of his reply is astounding. Rather than enter a legal debate on the validity of Mosaic law, Christ simply drew figures in the sand and asked those who had not sinned to cast the first stone. Gradually, the people so intent on punishment began to walk away, the older ones with more life lived (and therefore more mistakes made), being the first to leave. In this story, we see the recognition that when we focus on our own faults and weaknesses it helps to temper our tendencies to judge and punish others.

Another aspect of forgiveness is in the notion of letting go. Forgiveness means letting go the bitterness held against another, and ridding ourselves of the way that such bitterness affects our lives (much of what I discussed under the heading Letting Go, in Chapter 6, is also relevant here). Making a list of the injuries that have been inflicted by another and then watching it burn can be a useful symbolic method to ritualise letting go of the residual anger towards them. A third element in self-transcendence is that of making amends.

Making Amends

The focus here is not so much on the need to forgive others, but in helping the individual to forgive himself. In the early part of the book, I wrote of the reality that damaged people are not simply victims, but that they also have the capacity to hurt others. Very few damaged people have avoided hurting others out of their own dysfunction. Making amends is a useful step in healing some of the unfinished business of the past.

Making amends does not in many cases fix the hurts brought to other people. There are some hurts that are so great they will never be redeemed. Take, for example, a father or mother who through addiction or another major disorder has abused his or her children over a period of years. This, as we have seen earlier, is not an uncommon scenario. How can a recovering person make amends for this treatment of those children, who are now young adults deeply scarred by the experience? Nothing that a parent can do at this stage will change the reality of the lost years, of opportunity gone and of heartbreak. Making amends in this situation involves doing what is needed to help the individual reclaim some of what has been lost, to rebuild the relationships and to prevent any further damage. If, for instance, one of the children was unable to concentrate at school and underachieved as a result, then making amends might mean encouraging him or her to take a new interest in education and training, and to help support such an endeavour.

Another scenario consists of the child who on becoming a young adult who acts out her pain by way of addiction or some other compulsive behaviour. Making amends in this situation might involve discovering what help is available, and communicating the wish to do whatever is necessary to provide the individual with the resources she needs. These are the practical considerations, but the emotional elements of making amends include accepting responsibility for whatever pain has been caused, and getting to the point of apologising to the individual concerned. After that, it is up to the individual either to accept or reject it. In her healing process, there will come a time when she will be confronted with the choice to forgive.

Making amends can also be done in a symbolic way. This is of particular relevance when it is difficult or impossible directly to address the wrongs done to somebody, either because they would only be more hurt by any such attempts or because they are absent through separation or death. History is full of stories of people making ritual or symbolic attempts at redemption, and perhaps Joseph Conrad's novel Lord Jim portrays this process most insightfully. The novel's main character, Jim, exiles himself, and embarks on a journey of self-redemption, after an act of cowardice that betrays all his ideals. Whilst few of us need to engage in such dramatic action, most of us have some area of our lives where it would be healing to make amends. If we have hurt a life in some way, then we can choose to add something to the life of another in the particular area where we have caused the wound. Those who hurt children can perhaps find a way to help children. Those who, through greed and envy, have impoverished another might find a way to give to others. Those who have brought abuse into the life of another could find ways to help and support the carers of abuse victims. The 'how tos' of making amends are readily apparent for most people once they recognise the need to do so. It is very useful to consider that such attempts are best made with as little show as possible, thus avoiding the temptation to glory, or to feed off the goodwill most people have towards those who appear charitable.

Making amends in most situations will not heal the original hurt. Its focus must be on helping the agent of the hurt to learn from his mistakes and to become a better human being. That is the best that we can hope for any of us. Those badly wounded by others understand very clearly that attempts at redressing the wrong are often hollow and unsatisfactory, and that some hurts can never be redressed.

Self-Transcendence in the Absence of the Ego

Transcendent experience in the absence of the ego refers to a state of consciousness where the ego boundaries are lost and the person feels a sense of bliss and euphoria, and in most cases a sense of connection to forces beyond the self. Perhaps the greatest challenge facing modern life is that of the healthy integration of such transcendent experience into our technologically driven culture. More 'primitive' cultures have communal rituals available to people to assist in this part of their development. Dance, music, drumming and chanting are regularly used, sometimes with the assistance of hallucinogenic substances, such as peyote, hashish and ganja. In the absence of such rituals, certain modern versions are evolving in western societies, through the use of raves, ecstasy and alcohol as well as the growth of a variety of quasi-religious cults. These are dangerous equivalents, growing and expanding without any true understanding that they reflect real needs for mystical experiences as part of a healthy spiritual development.

Those who have heretofore been given the responsibility to cultivate and assist people in this part of human experience, namely the mainstream churches, have shown themselves to be bereft in this regard. This gap leaves the door wide open for people to engage in the cultivation of mystical experiences without understanding, control or supervision. As a result, addiction and self-destruction are exploding in the modern world. Mystical experiences become an escape route for many: from social alienation and deprivation, from inner emotional pain and from responsibility. This is instead of their healthy function, which is to nurture the soul, to bring security and peace and reaffirm the individual as to his or her place in the circle of life. It is therefore essential to understand that such transcendental experiences cannot replace the other areas of recovery, healing and growth that have been described thus far.

There is, as yet, no identifiable body of people in western society who tend to the needs of people by assisting this aspect of their spiritual growth. Rather, we see a phenomenon whereby various dubious individuals set themselves up as gurus. They present a variety of techniques for altering states of consciousness (many which are centuries old) to a naive and spiritually starving people, who accept and involve themselves uncritically, often with great damage to their lives. Teaching and guidance in the mystical aspects of spiritual growth is, therefore, urgently needed in the modern world. Whilst priests and pastors are the obvious people to carry out this function, they are, in many cases, unable to do so. This is because they have been taught much in terms of theology, are often kind hearted and generous, but their own spiritual development is uncared for as part of their training. Some, of course, are gifted in this realm, but in my opinion they are in the minority, and often have to struggle to hold on to their spiritual gifts - in spite of their training.

In the light of this reality, many therapists and counsellors find themselves confronted not with psychological problems, but with the suffering associated with a spiritual vacuum in alienated people. They too have been trained in one particular field, and are often out of their depth when it comes to spiritual matters. More than half a century ago, Victor Frankl called attention to this problem, but his voice has, to some extent, been lost. And those in the healing professions would do well to remember that we will not do a service to the healing of people as long as we, to use Victor Frankl's terms, 'tranquillise or analyse away' the real spiritual problems of people. Those who have some spiritual gifts, whether priests, pastors, counsellors or healers, need to cultivate and make them available to society at large.

Despite these overall difficulties, an individual can find some assistance in learning how to integrate mystical experiences into his or her spiritual growth. Certain areas of experience lend themselves to nurturing the soul through transcendent experience. Foremost among these are meditation, music, dance, visualisation and sexual intimacy.

Meditation

Meditation is recognised as one of the most effective methods of ego transcendence. There are many forms of meditation which are gentle and relaxing, and which have as their focus the emptying of one's mind from the distractions of everyday life. The exercises in these forms of meditation need not have any particular religious element, and can be accompanied by music to enhance the process of moving beyond the confines of the conscious ego. And one can use one's existing religious framework to understand such experiences. It is useful to have someone who can encourage and help with this process, and some counsellors are specialising in this area in response to the growing needs.

It is well recognised nowadays that these practices have their roots in the Eastern traditions of Buddhism and Hinduism. The most popular Westernized version now found under the rubric of mindfulness and courses are widely available both online and in class which can teach the basics of the techniques involved. Like everything else it is important to recognise both the strengths and weakness in any system that can be used to alter consciousness. Mindfulness and the practice of living in the now/present are particularly useful as a means of lowering stress and relieving anxiety and worry. As a lifestyle however it should come with a health warning insofar as it should be recognised that how we live in the present is radically important in terms of creating our future. Mindfulness can be seductive in suggesting that we practice watching the world, both internally and externally go by. And it can counsel against active engagement with life. That is a dangerous path to take.

Music, Dance and Visualisation

Certain types of music have for centuries been used to help transport people beyond the mundane into the mystical. The beat, rhythm and melody all combine on the listener's mind, creating the experience of a loss of ego boundaries, and a venture into beauty and euphoria. Beethoven, who knew so much of this experience, nicely summarised his view when he said that 'Music is the mediator between the spiritual and the sensual.' Currently, there is a massive growth in demand for a particular type of spiritually evocative music. Much of it is loosely termed new age, and listening to some of it I get a sense of a certain artificiality. There is a feeling that the artist has a goal in mind: to create another piece of mystical melody, and then stitches together a variety of riffs that have succeeded as a working formula. That said, there are others who seem to have a genuine, highly developed spirituality; it is as if they are already in the mystical world and bring their music back to us from it. Our own culture has, I believe, produced some of the best of this kind of music around.

Dance is another vehicle to bring us into mystical states. Unfortunately, the role of dance as part of spiritual ritual has been lost, and replaced by its use as a central part of the mating ritual. It has also become the territory of the young, and it is difficult to find opportunities to use expressive dancing in ways that are not to do with sexual pursuit or getting drunk. More recently, there has been some revival in the use of dance as a spiritual expression. This tends to be confined to weekend workshops. If dance is something that appeals to the reader, then it might be a useful experience to attend a dance workshop.

Visualisation refers to the use of the imagination to effect one's emotional or thinking state. We use visualisation constantly without being aware of it, and most of the time it is negative. We visualise bad things happening far more often than good. A useful example of positive visualisation is that of going on a journey to meet a loved one who has been away for some time. Sitting on the train or bus, a person will picture in his mind what she will look like when he arrives. Will her face seem the same? What will she be wearing? This ability to make pictures in one's mind is called visualisation, and it can be used as part of spiritual growth. Again, it may be useful to seek the help of someone who can lead people into a state of visualisation that involves the mystical experience of being surrounded by the love of God or the beauty of nature. These experiences nourish the soul, and allow the individual to return to the mundane and practical world refreshed and enlivened.

Sexual Intimacy

It may seem unusual to see sexuality discussed as part of spiritual growth. This is even more likely as a result of the ways that some of the social mores and views of sexuality have changed in recent times. We live in an age where sex has become a commodity. Bookshelves are lined with how-to manuals of all kinds, each heralding new and different techniques to enhance the physical operation of the sex act. 'Teach yourself good sex' videos are sold widely. Sexual toys and accessories are available to imitate, stimulate and penetrate various parts of the body in order to bring heightened pleasure and enjoyment. All of these have their place, and are useful in undermining the repressive attitudes to sexuality that have reigned in the minds of people throughout modern history.

There is, however, an implicit danger in seeing sex compartmentalised and packaged in this way, namely that the spiritual and mysterious elements of sexual intimacy can be lost. The key word here is intimacy. The spiritual element in sexual communication lies in the intimate relationship between two lovers. It does not operate to any great extent in casual sex, because there is no sense of truly 'knowing' and becoming lost in the other person through the experience of attachment and togetherness. For this to happen, there must be a great deal of trust and love operating between the people involved. And it is in this kind of relationship that there can be a source of deep spiritual as well as emotional and physical joy and celebration.

The human orgasm is a state of physical tension and release that is highly pleasurable. It also has the power to trigger a person into a state of mystical experience, where ego boundaries are collapsed and there is a deep emotional and spiritual connection to the partner. It is not surprising, then, that many people moan such religious expressions as 'Oh God' when they reach climax. Nor is it surprising that some people become sex addicts. I believe this occurs because the individual is chasing the mystical element of the experience through the pure physicality of the sex act. The experience they seeks is continually elusive They confuse the physical experience of orgasm with its spiritual correlates, not realising that the capacity to allow oneself into the mystical realm is not a matter of the number of sexual conquests, but rather a cultivation of one's own spirituality, which can then be enjoined with another in the sexual relationship.

In a love relationship, the spirituality of each partner can be nourished by paying attention to the spiritual and mystical elements of the sexual encounter. Doing so requires a sense of releasing oneself into the experience, and allowing the emotional as well as physical sensations to carry one along the path of self-forgetfulness and joy.

Summary

This chapter has considered the topic of spiritual growth, and its place in the process of healing and recovery. It has examined, albeit briefly, the area of cultivating a sense of the sacred, as well as seeking transcendental experiences that nourish the soul. It has also commented on the relationship between addiction and spirituality, a connection that in my opinion will become clearer over the next few years. In many ways, the contents of this chapter are best considered as signposts or possible pathways that can help the reader take an enlightened view of what is needed to assist in this part of development. It may also help an individual to provide an explanation, or frame, for understanding some spiritual experiences.

Afterword

There is a lot of content in this book and it is unrealistic to try to apply all the different forms of guidance advice and information at any one time. That would be overwhelming. Rather it is best used as a resource to dip into as time goes on and you encounter all the ups and downs and vagaries of life. There will be times when some aspects of the explanations and recommendations will be of particular relevance. Other times they may seem of little importance. Thus it is important to take from the above what you need when you need it. It would completely undermine the value and purpose of this book if it was to become a source of guilt, pressure or stress. In all the above there is one theme running through it, namely that you treat your life as important, and you treat yourself with dignity and respect.

Michael Hardiman. 2022

Bibliography

Beck, Aaron, Cognitive Therapy and the Emotional Disorders, London: Penguin Books 1991.

Bradshaw, John, The Family, Florida: Health Communications 1988.

Bradshaw, John, Healing the Shame that Binds You, Florida: Health Communications 1988.

Breggin, Peter, Toxic Psychiatry, London: Fontana 1993.

Campbell, Joseph, The Hero with a Thousand Faces, London: Fontana 1993.

Conrad, Joseph, Lord Jim, London: Penguin Books 1990.

Conroy, Pat, The Prince of Tides, London: Bantam 1988.

Dalrymple. T. Admirable Evasions. How Psychology Undermines Morality. New York. Encounter Books. 2015

De Mello, Anthony, Awareness, UK: Fount Paperbacks 1990.

Dobson, James, Dare to Discipline, Eastbourne: Kingsway 1970.

Dostoyevsky, F., Crime and Punishment, London: Penguin Books 1987.

Ellis, Albert, The Practice of Rational Emotive Behaviour Therapy, New York: Springer 1996.

Farrell, Bernard, I Do Not Like Thee, Doctor Fell, 1979.

Freud, Anna, The Ego and the Mechanisms of Defense, New York: International Universities Press 1946.

Freud, Sigmund, The Interpretation of Dreams, London: Pelican Books, 1976.

Furth, Greg, The Secret World of Drawings: Healing Through Art, US: Sigo Press 1989.

Gilbert, R. A., Casting the First Stone, The Hypocrisy of Religious Fundamentalism and its Threat to Society, Maine: Element 1993.

Grof, Christina, The Stormy Search for the Self, Understanding and Living with Spiritual Emergency, US:J.P. Tarcher 1993.

Hardiman, Michael, Children Under the Influence, Cork: Paragon Books 1993.

Hart, Josephine, Damage, US: Ivy Books 1992.

Hay, Louise, The Power is Within You, London: Eden Grove Editions 1991.

Ibsen, Henrik, The Wild Duck, Act V, cited in The Dust of Death by Os Guinness, Leicester: Inter-Varsity Press 1971.

Janov, Arthur, The Primal Scream, London: Abacus 1971.

Jung, Carl, Modern Man in Search of a Soul, London: Routledge, Kegan, Paul 1933.

Keenan, Brian, An Evil Cradling, London: Random House 1992.

Kilpatrick, W. K., Psychological Seduction: The Failure of Modern Psychology, Evesham: Arthur James 1985.

Kostenbaum, Peter, The New Image of the Person, New York: Greenwood Press 1978.

Lewis, C. S., Miracles, UK: Fount Paperbacks 1981

_________ , The Problem of Pain, UK: Fount Paperbacks 1981.

Marcel, Gabriel, The Philosophy of Existentialism, New Jersey: Citadel Press 1956.

Masson, Jeffrey, Against Therapy, London: Fontana 1990.

Miller, Alice, Banished Knowledge: Healing Childhood Injuries, London: Virago 1990.

Miller, Alice, For Your Own Good: Hidden Cruelty in Child Rearing and the Roots of Violence, London: Virago 1990.

Moore, Thomas, The Care of the Soul, London: Piatkus 1992.

Ofshe, Richard, Making Monsters: False Memories, Psychotherapy, and Sexual Hysteria, London: Deutsch 1995.

Peale, Norman. V The Power of Positive Thinking, London: Mandarin 1990.

Peck, M. Scott, Further Along the Road Less Travelled, New York: Simon and Schuster 1993.

Russell, Bertrand, A History of Western Philosophy, New York: Simon and Schuster 1972.

Sparks, Tav, The Wide Open Door: The Twelve Steps, Spiritual Tradition and the New Psychology, New York: Haselden 1993

Sugarman, Danny, Wonderland Avenue: Tales of Glamour and Excess, London: Sphere 1990.

Tournier, Paul, The Meaning of Persons, New York: Harper and Row 1968.

Tournier, Paul, The Person Reborn, New York: Harper and Row 1966.

Voltaire, F, Candide, New York Bantam 1993.

Wilde, Oscar, The Complete Works of Oscar Wilde, London: Collins 1989.

Whitfield, Charles, Healing the Child Within, Florida: Health Communications 1989.

Yalom, Irvin, Existential Psychotherapy, New York: Basic Books 1981.